# FITNESS.
# FOOD. FAITH.

## YOUR ETERNAL "WHY" FOR
## EVERLASTING RESULTS

KIM CLINKENBEARD CPT, FNS

Publishing services provided by 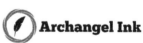 Archangel Ink

ISBN-13: 978-0-692-98958-6

# Contents

# PREFACE

This is *not* another self-help, weight loss, quick fix, or "my way is the best way" book.

I wrote this book because I want you to benefit from MY MISTAKES and SUCCESSES. If there was a program, diet, strategy or "solution," I tried it. If it was written, I read it. If it was a certification, I got it. If it was an infomercial, I probably bought it! I have shed blood, sweat, tears, and money for the possibility of a lean, healthy body.

I want to share with you how I fought my way back to health so you don't struggle for decades like me. I want you to know what it means to have ultimate health, balance, weight loss, fitness, peace, joy, and purpose and claim them for yourself!

It's a confusing maze of information and misinformation on health, wellness, diet, exercise, and how to obtain it all. In this book, I give you the tools needed to decipher between the fads and the truth through each of the three disciplines – Fitness, Food, and Faith. Knowledge is power. Use the information in this book to successfully make educated decisions about your health and what direction is best for *you*.

If you have found a nutrition plan (diet), exercise routine, program, or "way" to health that works for you, KEEP DOING

IT! Let this book encourage and motivate you to continue making progress. Use it to help fill in any gaps your current program may be lacking so you will be even *more* successful.

However, if you are lost, frustrated, sick, tired, ready to throw in the towel and "settle" for the way your health is now, KEEP READING. It's time to break free from the cycle of guilt, shame, doubt and defeat. I am sharing everything I have learned through decades of experience, education, and certifications as an expert in fitness and nutrition. And MY SECRET to EVERLASTING RESULTS—that has nothing to do with food or exercise!

The road to success is paved with mistakes. I hope that my experience, knowledge, and personal testimony help inspire you. You can live a life full of health, peace, joy, and purpose. Make the choice to learn a new way to optimal health. Believe anything is possible. Seek ultimate balance, health and wellness in your life. Understand why health is important, Biblically. Know God's purpose for you and your health. Find *your* Eternal "Why" and Everlasting Results.

*I will instruct you and teach you in the way you should go;*
*I will counsel you and watch over you.*
*Psalm 32:8*

# ACKNOWLEDGEMENTS

Thank you to my parents who ingrained in me an amazing work ethic. Thanks to my dad, who instilled a love for health and fitness in me by always leading by example. I owe all my creativity and adventurous spirit to my mom.

I owe a special thanks to my "circle of trust," who helped me through my health crises and continue to encourage me: Kim Southall, Claire Simons, Cheryl Green, Debbie Roland, Mariah Coy, and Laurie Wash.

I cannot express enough how thankful I am to all of those who sacrificed their time to help with this book by editing, reading, consulting, and praying: Tracy Clinkenbeard, Claire Simons, Hatel Patel, Kim Southall, Laurie Wash, Mary Ward, Cindy Nutter, Julie Allbright, Mary Hunt, and Joy Coleman.

Thank you to my sister-outlaws, Cheryl and Claire, who have inspired, taught and guided me in nutrition, and also share my passion for nutrition, health, and FOOD.

Finally, a big, special thanks to my amazing partner, best friend, and husband, Tracy. You always support every crazy idea and adventure I come up with. Thanks for kicking me in the booty when I need it and reigning me in when I get going too fast. Life is best with you!

# DEDICATION

For my grandma, Texana Chilton Cates. She was the strongest Christian woman I have ever known. God, family, exercise, and laughter were integral parts of her life until the very end of her 97 years. She loved and lived compassionately with a grateful heart. I only hope to live life as courageous and fully, while handling hardships as graciously as she did.

# HOW TO USE THIS BOOK

There is a common thread throughout each section of this book. The elements that contribute to a healthy body, mind, and spirit are interrelated and cannot be addressed separately. Some information presented in the *FITNESS SECTION* applies to the *FOOD SECTION*. Some of the information in the *FOOD SECTION* applies to the *FAITH SECTION*. Some of the information in the *FAITH SECTION* applies to everything, and so forth. My intention is that you can easily find answers, information, and recommendations quickly by the section headings. However, to fully grasp a clear and complete picture of ultimate health and wellness, you will want to read the entire book.

**USE THIS BOOK!** Highlight, write in the margins, dog ear pages. The scriptures and quotes scattered throughout are a special gift for you. They support the God-inspired writing. More importantly, they are included for you to meditate on, think about how they apply to your present circumstances, continue to connect you to God, and sometimes make you giggle. Use them in your special way.

There is a project I give my clients that I want to share with you, too. It's called a **"Pick Me Up Jar."** Here's how it works:

- Find any small container. It can be a mason jar, a decorative box, or something you make and decorate yourself. I use a small pretty tin I found at the craft store.
- Write down the scriptures and quotes scattered throughout this book. Add your own favorites, too.
- Fold them up and put them in your *"Pick Me Up Jar."*
- Whenever you're having a bad day, a bad thought (or string of them), feel like giving up on your goal, need motivation or a *Pick Me Up*, say a little prayer that God gives you the words you need to hear right now and pull out one of the strips of paper from your *"Pick Me Up Jar."*

I promise you will be blessed and refreshed if you give it a try! I'm amazed how the scripture or quote I draw from my *"Pick Me Up Jar"* is exactly what I need to hear. I encourage you to make yours soon and post pictures on my Facebook page @ getfitwithkimtoday.

I hope my testimony and the information you find here encourages, inspires, and educates you so you can find *your* eternal WHY and an everlasting healthy and happy life.

# FITNESS

"You will never out exercise a bad diet."
"Abs are made in the kitchen."
"You are what you eat."
"No pain, no gain."

These popular quotes are tossed around all the time in the fitness industry. While many of us jokingly reply, "Then, I'm 90% chocolate!" - or whatever the funny replies are- in truth, we are scared and overwhelmed by the fact that these statements are true.

**FACTS:**

- 3500 calories equal 1 pound of fat.

- To lose 1 pound, you must burn *more than* 3500 calories because you still have to eat.

Therefore, if it's impossible to lose weight by exercise alone and the only way to lose significant weight is to address your nutrition, then the big question is....

## WHY EXERCISE?

The benefits of exercise are indisputable. Scientific studies prove over and over that the more we move, the healthier we are and the longer we live.

"SITTING IS THE NEW SMOKING" was an attention-grabbing headline a few years ago. We know that smoking leads to cancer, heart disease, diabetes, and death. Research suggests that with every cigarette a person smokes, they take about 11 minutes off their life. Studies are showing the *same health risks* for those who spend most of their time *sitting*, whether at their desks or in front of the TV. However, instead of 11 minutes, it's been reported that for every HOUR a person SITS, *22 minutes* are taken off their life.

**STOP!** Let's read that again but make it a little more personal by adding the pronouns **I** and **MY**.

FOR EVERY HOUR **I** SIT, 22 MINUTES
ARE TAKEN OFF **MY** LIFE.

Did that get your attention? It resonated with me, and I've never been one to spend much time sitting, in part because I don't have a desk job. However, most working adults *do* have a job where much of their day is sitting behind a desk or the wheel of a vehicle. Not only are adults suffering from the effects of a sedentary lifestyle, so are our children.

Obesity is on the rise. It's predicted that by 2030, 51% of the American population will be obese, and 60% or more of them will have diabetes or pre-diabetes. On the flip side, studies show that incorporating *just 15-30 minutes of exercise a day* can delay the onset of obesity related diseases. Add nutritional changes to a well-rounded exercise program, and obesity related diseases can be *reversed.*

**A well-rounded exercise program will help you with the following.** I've included a translation in case the medical reasons aren't enough:

➤ Appetite Control

*Translation: APPETITE CONTROL!!! You will no longer feel the need to constantly stand in front of the fridge in hopes that something "good" to eat will magically appear since the last time you looked, which in turn will save you money on your electric bill.*

➢ Better Sleep

*Translation: NO MORE BAGS under your eyes = save money on makeup and facial creams.*

➢ Maintain a Healthy Weight

*Translation: Look good in the mirror and fit into that swimsuit you've passed by at the department store 10 times this summer.*

➢ Lower Blood Pressure, Resting Heart Rate, and Bad Cholesterol

*Translation: Get the doctor off your back and reduce or eliminate medications.*

➢ Reduce Stress and Anxiety

*Translation: Less road rage, better mood, a positive outlook, and more friends.*

➢ Increase Energy

*Translation: You get more checked off the "honey do" list and have more free time for fun stuff and date night!*

➢ Strong Muscles and Bones

*Translation: You won't get trapped under the 50-lb. bag of dog food that falls on you when loading it into your SUV.*

➢ Stronger Immune System

*Translation: Less time off work, so you will keep that job you love, which will pay for that vacation where you can wear your new swimsuit.*

➢ Better Digestion

*Translation: You don't look like you swallowed a basketball by mid-afternoon.*

Joking aside, both smoking and sedentary lifestyles accelerate disease and lead to a shorter life span. Not to mention, a poorer quality of life. The fact is, exercise does improve health and increase longevity and quality of life.

If those reasons weren't enough, exercise also supports weight loss efforts by building lean muscle which in turn, burns more calories. Exercise makes our hearts and lungs stronger, making our bodies more efficient and burn more calories at rest.

I know, I know. I just got the eye roll. All that's great, but it's still not enough to motivate us to exercise! So, now what?

## WE NEED TO START LOOKING AT EXERCISE DIFFERENTLY.

Proverbs 4:23 says, *"Be careful how you think, your life is shaped by your thoughts."* If you change your PERSPECTIVE - the way you look at things you want to change - then tasks become easier, life becomes less overwhelming and more manageable, and the impossible becomes possible. [1]

Exercise is like brushing our teeth. A "non-negotiable." We never skip brushing our teeth; unless we are sick or in the hospital. When healthy and able, we brush our teeth at least once a day, *no matter what.* Exercise falls into the same category. We

---

1  Your beliefs become your thoughts, your thoughts become your words, your words become your actions, your actions become your habits, your habits become your values, your values become your destiny. – Mahatma Gandhi

should do *purposeful* exercise *every single day.* NO MATTER WHAT.[2] Exercise must become a habit we DO NOT break.[3]

God designed our bodies to be active and moving to work properly. When you're moving; joints are lubricated, muscles are strong and flexible, bones are dense and strong, the heart and lungs are strong and efficient (blood flows easier resulting in lower blood pressure and heart rate), and the digestive system and bowels work properly and efficiently. We are designed to move, PERIOD.

That doesn't mean you have to live at the gym and exercise hardcore for two hours a day, seven days a week. You can incorporate movement and exercise into your workday so, *cumulatively,* you are moving throughout the day and not sedentary for more than an hour or two at a time.

The number one focus for my new clients is learning to view *exercise as the means to live the lifestyle they want to live for the rest of their lives.*

> *If you view EXERCISE as the way to BURN CALORIES*
> *and LOSE WEIGHT,*
> *you will ALWAYS STRUGGLE with MOTIVATION*
> *and with WEIGHT LOSS.*

When you have the mindset that you can *eat what you want* and *exercise to burn it off,* you will be *nutritionally deficient* and *always chasing after* a healthy, lean body - *but never getting one.* You take two steps forward and one step back. Personally,

---

2   Good habits are worth being fanatical about. – John Irving

3   So much of what we do every single day is the result of habits that we have formed over time. – Joyce Meyer

my goal is to maintain a level of fitness that allows me to do any physical activity that I want to do at any time. I never want to think to myself, "Oooh, I don't know if I can go skiing this weekend because I'm not sure I'm in shape enough to ski! I need at least a month to get in shape." I want the freedom that comes with being in a *constant state of physical fitness.*

YOGA? RUNNING? WEIGHT LIFTING? CROSS FIT? ZUMBA? AEROBICS? CYCLING?

## WHICH FORM OF EXERCISE IS BEST to support your health AND boost your METABOLISM?

The list of workouts is as endless as the opinions of which style burns the most amount of fat, raises metabolism, and is best for getting in shape. So, the answer is:

THE WORKOUT YOU WILL DO **CONSISTENTLY**
IS THE BEST ONE FOR YOU.[4]

**The #1 thing for success in an exercise or nutrition program is to be CONSISTENT and PERSISTENT**.[5] If you are inconsistent in your workouts, all you are going to do is make yourself SORE and EXTREMELY HUNGRY, damaging your metabolism in the process. (Although, the damage *is* reversible with consistency in nutrition and exercise.) *Exercising for an hour, two or three times a week, and being primarily sedentary the rest of the week, will harm your health.* You are not going to see the benefits of exercise listed above unless you *consistently* exercise

---

4   The only bad workout is the one that didn't happen. – Unknown

5   We become what we repeatedly do. – Sean Covey

*every* day. Not every workout needs to be long or intense. Walking for 30 minutes on your non-workout days will help with the benefits, but *you must be intentionally active every day to reap the benefits of exercise.*

Look at it this way; **If you put in 10% effort, you will get a 10% return.**[6] The more you put in, the more you get out. I don't know about you, but I don't have a spare minute to waste. If I'm going to set aside the time to change clothes, drive to the gym, sweat, drive home, shower, and get dressed *again,* then I want a great return for that effort. When I exercise, I put 100% into the workout so I get the most return from my effort. This applies to all aspects of life, not just exercise and diet.[7]

**Your workouts should be designed to SUPPORT your lifestyle and goals.**

If you have no interest in running a triathlon, there is no need to spend hours on the bicycle, running, or swimming. If your favorite hobby is playing golf, add workouts to your schedule (3-4 times a week) that will improve your golf game. You are more likely to do the workouts that improve the activities you enjoy.

If you enjoy your workouts, you will continue doing them. You won't fall in love with every hard-core workout that's necessary to improve your fitness. But if you know that it's going to help

---

6  2 Corinthians 9:6 "Remember this: Whoever sows sparingly will also reap sparingly, and whoever sows generously will also reap generously."

7  Galatians 6:7-8 "Do not be deceived: God cannot be mocked. Whatever a man sows, he will reap in return. The one who sows to please his flesh, from the flesh will reap destruction; but the one who sows to please the Spirit, from the Spirit will reap eternal life."

you continue doing what you love, then you will be more willing to put the effort into it.

**For those of you whose hobbies consist of watching TV, sewing, reading, or other sedentary activities, you must find some type of exercise you will do.**

If you DO NOT incorporate some form of physical activity into every day, you will:

| A sedentary lifestyle leads to: |
| --- |
| » *Heart disease* |
| » *Osteoporosis* |
| » *Diabetes* |
| » *Arthritis* |
| » *Irritable bowel syndrome* |
| » *Colitis* |
| » *Insomnia* |
| » *Alzheimer's* |
| » *Dementia* |
| » *Cancer* |

- shorten your lifespan
- have a poor quality of life
- accelerate diseases related to a sedentary lifestyle

Eventually, lack of exercise will disrupt your ability to SIT comfortably due to leg swelling, sciatica, and back pain, which will make your hobbies less enjoyable at best.

Find some form of physical activity - even if it's walking - that you can do and enjoy. The movement will help you eliminate water retention, back pain, sciatica, and detoxify your body. You will find that you are happier and more productive. Not to mention the added years to your life.

# DEALING WITH THE "I DON'T WANT TO's"

**What if you don't *FEEL* like working out today? When do you take a day off?**

Do I *feel* like working out every day? Absolutely, NOT! I don't *feel* like doing a lot of things: making my bed, taking out the trash, driving the speed limit, picking up dog poo. (I NEVER *feel* like picking up dog poo!) However, when you do these necessary "evils," so to speak, at bare minimum, you feel a sense of accomplishment. Not to loop picking up dog poo in with exercise, *but* you will reap even more benefits from doing all the above, consistently, whether you *feel* like it or not. **Don't base your health on your feelings at the time.** There are consequences to your actions and inactions.

EVERY time I have worked out, even though I didn't *feel* like it, I have felt more energetic, better about myself, and accomplished. PERIOD. On the contrary, every time I skipped a workout because I didn't *feel* like doing it, I partook in another bad behavior -like eating half a pie- which left me feeling defeated, fatigued, sick, and plagued with the negative self-talk and thoughts that seem to follow. Does this mean every workout must be some Olympic measure of athleticism? NO WAY! Even if you only do 15 minutes of intense exercise (or just walk), you will feel so much better for it. I promise![8]

---

8  Our daily decisions and habits have a huge impact upon both our levels of happiness and success. – Shawn Anchor

## STRATEGIES TO HELP YOU THROUGH THE "I DON'T WANT TO's":

➤ **Get dressed** (in your workout clothes!) and **LEAVE THE HOUSE.**

- ○ Because I train clients at my house, exercising on those days is easy for me. If I don't have clients, I will find any and every excuse to get "too busy" or distracted from finishing a workout – the phone rings or the dryer buzzes. If I go to the gym, I'm more likely to start, and finish, my work out on those days.

➤ **Keep a consistent workout time.**

- ○ If I normally workout at 9:30 am, I will keep that same time on the days I have the "I don't want to's." I know that if I put off exercising until later in the day with the hope of eventually *feeling* like it, I will NEVER actually do it. Putting off a workout has NEVER worked in my favor.

➤ **Make a deal with yourself.**

- ○ I'll only do a hard 15 minutes.
- ○ I'll do 5 sets of intervals within that time frame.
- ○ It's only 15 minutes! I can do that!
- ○ I have almost always ended up doing longer (or at least harder) workouts than planned when I showed up with the "deal" that I'd only *have* to do 15 minutes. Once you get the blood pumping, the oxygen flowing, and the feel-good chemicals released in the brain, you will feel better and generally do more than intended.

➢ **Be OK with what you can give that day!**

- ○ Some days are just harder than others. Cut yourself a break occasionally if you are consistently giving 100%. Being consistent in your workouts *every* day will be **cumulatively** better for your health, fitness, and goals than only working out 2-3 times a week (no matter how long those workouts are). **The cumulative result is what matters most.** Plus, it will deeply ingrain within you the habit of exercising. [9]

➢ **Be GRATEFUL** that you have a capable, functioning body that allows you to exercise!

- ○ This is not a liberty everyone has. We tend to take our health and bodies for granted. Don't make this mistake.

➢ Understand that **you DO HAVE THE TIME AND ABILITY** to exercise **TODAY**.

- ○ No one is promised tomorrow. We have no idea what tomorrow will bring: we could get sick, someone could get injured and need us, our car could breakdown, or work might interfere. A million things could happen to rob you of your exercise time. A consistent workout schedule will help you keep your fitness and health when "life" happens and you *must* skip a workout.

➢ **Find your "WHY" and LIVE it!**

- ○ If you know *"WHY"* you are exercising, then you will draw strength and motivation from that goal/reason on the days you don't *feel* like exercising. Or eating

---

9   Habits change into character. -Ovid

right for that matter. More on your "WHY" in the FAITH SECTION!

## THE ONLY TIME IT'S OK TO TAKE A DAY OFF IS:

- If you are sick with fever, nausea, diarrhea, or some other major illness/symptom.

  Here's one of my favorite rhymes to help remember this:

  *"If it's in your head, get out of bed. If it's in your chest, stay home and rest."*

- If you are over-trained, i.e. overly stressed physically to the point you are getting injured and/or sick.

- If you are overly stressed mentally/emotionally to the point you are not sleeping and are getting sick frequently.[10]

  If you have family commitments interfering with your workout that day: vacation, wedding, family member hospitalized, graduation etc.

- ALTHOUGH, most of the time, good time-management will allow you to squeeze in a 15-minute, intense workout, no matter what the conflict is.

**Taking just ONE day off because you just don't *feel* like exercising WILL lead to taking several days off and ultimately quitting exercising all together.** Or at best, you will be very sporadic with your workouts, which will only make you miserably SORE and HUNGRY!

---

10 Psalm 71:16a "I will walk in the strength of the Lord."

# HOW MUCH TIME DO YOU NEED TO SPEND EXERCISING EACH DAY?

It depends on a couple of factors:

## 1. Your lifestyle: are you predominately SEDENTARY or ACTIVE?

- Does your job require that you sit or drive for several hours a day?
- Is your commute long, requiring you to be in the car for an hour or more each day?
- Does your "after work schedule" involve more sitting with kids doing homework or watching TV to unwind?

If your answer is **"YES"** to any or all of these questions, then you will need to spend **more** time exercising to reach any significant health benefit and offset the time you spend sitting.

I know this sounds daunting when you are already exhausted by the time you get off work, but **there's good news!** Especially for those who do not have a lot of spare time or resources to devote to exercising or joining a gym.

Many studies have found that **short bouts of exercise throughout the day** have the **same benefits as continuous workouts.** This means that if you are short on time and it works better for you to split your routine into several short workouts throughout the day, don't worry that you won't burn as many calories or get good results.

**Incorporating short bursts of exercise (5-10 minutes) throughout the day will recharge your brain, rev up your**

**metabolism, and give you the extra energy you need to finish your day *without* caffeine, energy drinks, and sugar.**

Set your alarm, grab your coworkers and get a quick workout in mid-day. You don't have to change clothes or even break a sweat!! Do what you can within your fitness level and capabilities. If you don't feel comfortable or cannot do certain exercises, then just move – march in place, dance, do jumping jacks. If you can't do 10 push-ups (yet), then just do one. If you can't do a squat, then try getting out of your chair without using your hands. (In fact, everyone should try that exercise. And those of us over 40, try it without making the "Uhhh" sound! Ha ha.) *Just try to improve every week.* Even if you are already exercising consistently, this is a great way to get a little extra! **The key is to find a schedule that works for you.** [11]

> **NOTE:** The only time to worry about continuous exercise versus short bouts of exercise is if you are training for a specific competition or sport where you may need continuous exercise to prepare your body for that activity – like running a marathon, playing hockey or soccer, or ultra-endurance cycling.

For the average person exercising for weight management or control, stress release, and overall health, splitting up their workouts throughout the day can mean the difference between life and death - literally.

---

11    If you really want to do something, you'll find a way. If you don't, you'll find an excuse. – Jim Rohn

**Here are a few suggestions to help you incorporate exercise throughout your day:**

➤ Set your phone alarm for strategic times during the day (for example 10:00am, 2:00pm, 4:00pm, and 7:00pm). This will depend on your level of fitness and work schedule. If you're afraid your coworkers will think you've finally "lost it," make them do this with you!

➤ Pick 2-4 different exercises that require little or no equipment like squats, jumping jacks, push-ups, or going up and down the stairs.

➤ Depending on your schedule, set your timer for 3-10 minutes. Perform 10-20 repetitions of each exercise you chose for the duration of the time allotted. You can repeat the same exercises and time, or switch it up. The combinations are endless.

➤ Purchase an over-the-door pull-up bar for the house/office and do a few pull-ups every time you want to grab that energy drink or candy bar. Or every time you pass by it.

➤ Start an office push-up/pull-up contest – see how many push-ups/pull-ups you can do in 1 minute every week. (Prizes always make this a little more appealing.)

I don't know how many times my workout consisted of having a dance party with my nephew and dog while doing laundry and other house chores. It still counts! **You don't have to go to the gym to get a good workout.** Be creative and use what you have around you to make a workout. Even skipping down the street in intervals is a GREAT workout! If you haven't skipped since you were 7 years old, I highly recommend going outside and trying it! It's surprisingly hard. Plus, there is absolutely no possible way to stay in a bad mood and NOT smile while skipping! If you feel silly, then grab your kids, or the neighbor kids – get permission first - and get them to skip with you. It's something that also helps the kiddos get their exercise, since childhood obesity is a fast-rising epidemic in our country. You can turn anything into a game with a little creativity and imagination. The possibilities for incorporating activity into your day are endless.

**TIP:** TIMING IS ESSENTIAL. Make the most of the time you have.

The first thing I noticed at the gym this morning was how "busy" it was. I put busy in quotes because it looked like a bad zombie movie with most of the people wandering around with blank expressions on their faces. Don't get me wrong. There were a few who obviously had a routine they were doing, but most exercisers were plodding along on a treadmill or sitting on a piece of equipment. And I'm not talking about the first-time exercisers, either. I'm talking about the same people I've seen at various gyms over the past 20+ years. They do the same thing year after year and *look* the same year after year. The worst part? They were still wandering around when I left - 45 minutes later! I don't think they had even broken a sweat.

People get stuck in a routine for many reasons:

    a.  they are afraid to change it

    b.  they don't know what or how to change

    c.  they don't see the need to change it

Consequently, they go day after day, year after year, never getting results, and spending hours of their day in the gym in the process. I love the gym and exercising, or I would not have made it my profession. However, the *last* place I want to spend my FREE TIME is in the gym.

**Try this technique this week to jump start your routine – OLD or NEW – to make the most of your time:**

Set your timer or watch for 30 minutes. Or for those of you who feel like you must spend hours in the gym to make it worthwhile; set it for *HALF the time you normally workout*. Make it a point to fit your routine into the allotted time frame. This may mean you take fewer or NO rest breaks. Or you may realize a few more exercises need to be added. Either way, I promise you will get a *HARDER workout in LESS time*.

The 2nd factor that determines HOW MUCH TIME you need to spend exercising:

## 2. The state of your PHYSICAL and MENTAL HEALTH at any given time.

- If you are healthy, then the sky is the limit.
  - Pick an activity you enjoy and work your way up to an advanced level of exercise.
  - If you want to complete or compete in an ultra-endurance sport (like triathlon and marathon) then form a plan and train to reach that goal.

- If you are suffering from a chronic disease like arthritis or recovering from an injury, surgery, or illness; then you need to take it easy until you are fully healthy and recovered. Resume exercise according to your doctor's recommendations.

- If you are going through a hardship – death, divorce, a loss, move, new job, marriage, pregnancy, etc.- then exercise will definitely help. However, more is not always better when you are overly stressed in other areas of life. By all means, exercise and keep active. Exercise will help reduce stress, boost your mood, reduce depression, increase mental clarity, and lower blood pressure. However, OVER-EXERCISING (more than hour a day) to "DEAL" with stresses in your life will do more HARM than good. It will lead to overtraining, injury, weakened immune system, illness, fatigue, depression, and more. If you need help "DEALING" with a high stress situation in your life, seek professional counseling. Use exercise to keep a level of fitness during this season in your life, NOT (solely) as a coping mechanism to avoid your problems, struggles, or life itself.

## MY STORY

In 2012, I hit a physical and mental mountain. (I was going to write "stumbling block," but that just didn't do it justice.)

I had neither the physical energy nor the mental capacity to finish a conversation much less complete a workout that was more than 20 minutes long (which included walking the dog for 15 of those minutes). I couldn't exercise for more than 2-3 days a week. Getting three days of exercise in each week was a good week. This lasted for almost three years!

I distinctly remember the week I was finally able to exercise for 30 minutes, for five days! It was a huge milestone for me.

I had literally gone from racing 70.3 Ironman Triathlons (1.2-mile swim, 56-mile bike, 13.1-mile run) to not being able to get off the couch and train clients for more than 1-2 hours at a time. My day consisted of getting out of bed after maybe two hours of sleep, going to the gym to train clients for two hours, coming home and sitting on the couch until I had to train clients in the afternoon. I didn't even want to think about cooking supper. Most days I was too exhausted to shower. (Of course, when you're just sitting on the couch, you don't get too terribly dirty. Thank goodness!)

Only a couple of months before, I had almost completely recovered from reconstructive foot surgery 18 months prior. I was training several clients, working out every day, running up to six miles three times a week, and getting back in race shape.

Suddenly, I got a stress fracture in my "new" foot. **RED FLAG #1.** (Now, some of you keyed in on the fact that being so exhausted I couldn't function **was not my first RED FLAG.** One would think it would register with me, but honestly, I thought I was sick with Mono or something.) I went back to my foot surgeon and physical therapist for x-rays, bone density scans, and more physical therapy.

Unfortunately, **after 9 months**, my stress fracture was still not healing! **RED FLAG #2.** My workouts suffered because I was back in a walking boot and using crutches. I was still not sleeping. I couldn't remember anything. I would leave the room mid-sentence and do something else not realizing I hadn't finished the conversation. I was moody and irritable –

a female version of Jekyll and Hyde. I could hear myself snap at my husband for no reason, but I just couldn't stop the crazy train from leaving the station. If you're shouting "YES, sister! I hear you! This is me!"— let me assure you that you are NOT crazy, and you are NOT alone.

While my nutrition was spot on, I was still gaining weight. My hair was falling out by the fistfuls, and EVERY DAY I felt like I had just run 2 marathons before I even got out of bed. **RED FLAGS #3, 4, 5, 6, 7, 8, 9, and 10.**

My job was suffering. Forget going to church regularly, or anywhere else. My friendships suffered. My marriage was strained; although, now, we can see this brought us closer together. This amazing man of mine stood by me even when I was awful to him. He understood that I was sick and SCARED. He was constantly saying, "We will figure this out. I promise we will find the solution and you will get healed!" I will confess there were times his optimism really ticked me off! Looking back, I'm so thankful that he was bringing light into a very dark situation. I thank God every day for him.

### SIDE BAR: MEN, I'M TALKING DIRECTLY TO YOU:

IF YOUR WIFE OR LOVED-ONE IS GOING THROUGH HORMONAL CHANGES/DIFFICULTIES, whether diagnosed or not, please continue to encourage and support her. It *will* get better.

MEN NEED SUPPORT, TOO. This is hard stuff! I keep telling my husband, Tracy, that he needs to start a men's support group for those helping their women through this stage of life. You may not like to talk through your problems, but I recommend it. Contact my husband! He's happy to talk with you.

Women going through hormone-related issues are *scared*. They need reassurance that you are not leaving them; they will get better; and that you think they're desirable!! It may sound trite, but what I needed most from my husband was to know that he still found me sexy and attractive because I felt everything BUT sexy and attractive.

Here's one scripture you can repeat to your loved-one during the hardest times:

*Romans 5: 2b-5 "And we rejoice in the hope of the glory of God. Not only so, but we also rejoice in our sufferings, because we know that suffering produces perseverance; perseverance, character; and character, hope. And hope does not disappoint us, because God has poured out His love into our hearts by the Holy Spirit, whom He has given us."*

There are so many encouraging scriptures for both of you. This is the one Tracy recited to me, constantly. He literally wrote on my bathroom mirror, "Endeavor to Persevere!"

Hang in there. After getting through the hard times together, you will be stronger together because of it. Here is a scripture for you to hold on to:

*2 Corinthians 4:17 "For our light and momentary troubles are achieving for us an eternal glory that far outweighs them all."*

Take time together to read these verses tonight. They comforted us.

*2 Corinthians 4:16-18 and Romans 8:18, 28-29a.*

## BACK TO MY STORY

My relationships were suffering. My emotions were all over the place. I felt like I had NO control over anything, including my thoughts. The last punch in the stomach was when I was told, "There was nothing structurally wrong with my foot to cause the stress fracture. Something was wrong, hormonally, to cause my stress fracture."

My foot surgeon recommended I see a doctor and test my hormone levels. At the time, this was NOT good news to me! I was hoping my foot could be surgically repaired. I did NOT want to find MORE health problems.

However, my surgeon was instrumental in my TOTAL healing, not only by rebuilding my foot, but also by guiding us to find the TRUTH about my health. (He is one of the best Christian men I know, and we are honored to call him friend and brother in Christ.)

After 9 months of dealing with a stress fracture that would not heal, dealing with the rest of the nightmarish symptoms, endless research, and countless conversations, I finally went to my OBGYN and requested they test EVERYTHING. (A list of recommended lab tests is available on page 236.)

What the tests revealed lead me down a path of physical, mental, and spiritual healing and transformation that I would have never imagined, but would not trade for anything now.

*"For it is by grace you have been saved, through faith – and this not from yourselves, it is the gift of God – not by works, so that no one can boast. For we are God's workmanship, created in Christ Jesus to do good works, which God prepared in advance for us to do." Ephesians 2:8–10*

## KEY COMPONENTS TO A WELL-BALANCED EXERCISE PROGRAM

The human body comes in many shapes, sizes, and abilities. While some have short, strong muscles that help them jump high and sprint fast, others have long, lean muscles that help them endure long distances. We are not all created equal in that respect, but what we do share, which does *not* differ between body types are:

### FIVE KEY ELEMENTS that help every BODY function at its optimal best:

1) **STRENGTH TRAINING:** Strength training is often thought of as strictly lifting weights (and for building big muscles for body building). This is a common misconception, especially among women. Strength training *does* need to involve weight bearing activities to improve muscle tone and size, bone density, joint stabilization and overall strength. But it does NOT have to involve lifting heavy weights. Although weights should be incorporated into every training program, using your own body weight produces amazing results. Adding plyometrics, medicine balls, planks, push-ups, pull-ups, squats, sprints, and

lunges to your routine will dramatically improve overall strength and appearance.

2) **CARDIOVASCULAR TRAINING:** Cardiovascular training (commonly referred to as "cardio") involves working both the Cardiovascular (heart) and Respiratory (lungs) Systems. Cardio is typically something people either love or hate and subsequently over-do or over-look.

Runners will do nothing *except* run, while body builders will *neglect* cardio altogether thinking it will "eat their muscle tissue" - which is NOT TRUE, by the way. The fact is, your heart is also a muscle that needs training to handle the loads of strength training, core training, and everyday life and stress. Cardio training does this for you. Don't worry. Training for a marathon is not necessary to reap the benefits. Incorporating cardio exercises such as biking, running, walking, rowing, circuit training, or even jumping jacks into your strength or core workouts will reap *significant* cardiovascular endurance.

I mix it up by combining core, strength, and cardio into a SINGLE workout. Eliminating or reducing rest periods between sets will also make a strength training workout more cardiovascular. If you are crunched for time, a combination workout is the way to go!

3) **CORE TRAINING:** While you can't bench press your way across a finish line, a strong back, chest and shoulders will help maintain your proper form while running, biking, skipping, (or for some of us, crawling) across it. Without a strong cardio-respiratory system, you won't be able to complete an intense strength training session. A strong core *will* help support your posture and spine in *every*

activity you choose including carrying grandkids and putting boxes on the top shelf. Without a strong core, your strength and cardio training efforts will plateau quickly, or you can be injured.

Your core is comprised of more than abdominal training (i.e. crunches). To develop a strong core, it's essential to incorporate balance and stability training. Other muscle groups included in your core that tend to be overlooked are low back extensors, pelvic floor, glutes, and mid traps. You can contact me directly at www.getfitwithkimtoday.com for help designing a complete exercise program.

4) **FLEXIBILITY TRAINING:** Ahhh, my nemesis. I will admit that flexibility is the element that gives me the most trouble. I don't mind gutting it up in the gym or riding the bike for five hours, but stretching gets put on the back burner all too often. Or *used to be* put on the back burner. Over the years (and many injuries) I have gained a new respect for flexibility. Bodies will NOT function in a chronically tight state. Eventually, injury will occur, sometimes requiring surgery.

I find traditional stretching techniques like static stretching boring. Science has proven traditional methods of static stretching decrease strength. Researchers at NASM (National Academy of Sports Medicine) recommend other forms of dynamic stretching to be the *"most effective at improving flexibility in athletes."*

There are other more beneficial (and fun, I might add) ways to gain flexibility, including SMR (self-myofascial release), dynamic stretching, active stretching, Pilates, yoga, and Tai Chi. Incorporate flexibility into your exercise routine and reap the rewards of this patience-required skill. My workouts are designed to include dynamic flexibility throughout. It's the most effective and time efficient way to gain flexibility.

5) **REST** is the final element to a well-rounded exercise program and healthy body. Some have rest down to an art form – doing more *rest* than anything else. Others get anxious if they miss even *one* workout, never taking a day off. We should aim for a BALANCE in our exercise routine. Allowing a little recovery not only lets muscles rebuild and become stronger, but gives joints a break and provides a *mental* rest.

Without the necessary physical and mental rest, we burn out and often quit exercising. If you're having difficulty moving past a plateau or finding motivation to continue exercising, re-evaluate your schedule. Do you have a rest day? If not, start there. Perhaps you have *too many* rest days. In this case, add variety to your workout routine by incorporating one of the other elements you may be neglecting.

People tend to gravitate to ONE of these FIVE ELEMENTS over the others depending on what comes naturally. Focusing on sport-specific training is a must to succeed at your sport, but neglecting the other four elements will eventually hinder your performance. Even if you are only exercising for your health and lifestyle, attention to strength, cardio, core, flexibility, and rest will change not only your physical ability, but also the way you move and feel *all the time.*

# EXERCISE MYTHS

Everyone has a philosophy on how and when to exercise. It can get confusing, to say the least. Below are a few common myths, debunked.

1) Lifting weights vs. cardio: one is better than the other.

   ○ **FALSE.** They are different and both necessary for weight loss and overall health. Doing only one form of exercise is like eating only meat – you need a variety of foods, including veggies, to live a long, healthy life.

2) Quickly lifting weights counts as cardio.

   ○ **FALSE.** Yes, it's true: H.I.I.T. (High Intensity Interval Training) is the best option for exercise for those with limited amounts of time and should be included in *every* workout program. However, if not structured correctly, they will leave you over-trained. H.I.I.T. workouts should not be done every day. If you are quickly lifting weights as a substitute for cardio training (meaning the tempo is fast, which sacrifices form), you are setting yourself up for major injuries. (See the section on H.I.I.T. workouts for more information about the importance of why and how to do them.)

3) If you don't feel completely exhausted or puke after a workout, you didn't exercise hard enough.

   ○ **FALSE.** This is probably the biggest myth out there! Somehow, we have gotten the idea that exercise should be torturous, when in fact, exercise should make you feel GOOD! It *should* relieve stress, muscle tightness, fatigue, excess water weight, and fat. You *should* feel ENERGIZED after a workout - even a very challenging workout. Exercising to the extreme of puking should never be encouraged. Not only is it NOT fun (and makes your breath stink!), it's also dangerous.

4) You should stretch and warm up BEFORE exercise.

- **TRUE & FALSE.** The fact is, our bodies is a warm 98.6° all the time. What exactly are we supposed to "warm up" to? To prepare your body for exercise, begin slowly for the first few minutes with dynamic stretches built into your workout. This qualifies as "warming up" and is the best way to gain functional flexibility without adding unnecessary time and movements to your workout. You will not only save time but also be shocked at how much flexibility and strength you will gain *quickly*. And did I mention that you will save a lot of time?!

5) You will burn muscle if:

- You do cardio before weights. **FALSE**
- You do only cardio. **FALSE**
- You do too much cardio. **FALSE**

Your personal goals determine the order of your workouts – cardio vs. weights. Save the most energy for the workout that's your PRIMARY FOCUS that day. I recommend doing cardio and weights on separate days. However, if you are competing in ultra-endurance sports like triathlon, marathon, soccer, basketball, etc. then you will be doing cardio six days a week. In that case, do a split workout -

cardio in the morning and weights at least three hours later. The same is true for body building or power lifting.

Can we agree that sprinting is very cardiovascular? It's also going to build *significant* muscle mass. So, to say that "cardio" burns muscle is just silly. Have you seen the Olympic Sprinters? Your heart is also a muscle, and needs to be strengthened. If you are doing "quality" cardio, you will burn fat and calories, as well as build functional muscle.

If your cardio sessions are long and slow, you will not gain the health benefits or weight loss, and will end up extremely hungry! If structured correctly, cardio will help build muscle, reduce weight and excess water (bloating), raise metabolism, and regulate hunger (insulin sensitivity).

6) You burn more calories if you exercise first thing in the morning before you eat.

   ◦ **FALSE.** This is a personal thing. If you are a 5 a.m.-er, go for it! Personally, I can't get a good workout at 5 a.m. That's prime sleep time for me. Pick a time of day when YOU are *most motivated* and have the *most energy* to workout. Then, you will burn the *most calories....*

   As far as exercising on an empty stomach goes - that's also a personal preference. Because of specific training for 70.3 Ironman Triathlons (which takes me 6 hours to complete), I can eat WHILE I exercise just fine. Some people get sick if they don't have a little something in their tummy before a workout. Play around with eating something light (like 1/2 an apple or 1 slice toast with a little peanut butter for example)

30-45 minutes before your next workout and see how you feel. If you are good with exercising on an empty stomach, go for it! Let hunger and how you feel during your workouts be your guide.

If structured correctly, both cardio and strength/weight training will help you reach any goal you have. **The take away is:** QUALITY workouts will give you the health and results you desire. Everyone needs to include BOTH cardio and strength training with dynamic flexibility into their regimen for *overall, balanced* **health benefits.** Seek help from a certified fitness professional in structuring a safe and effective workout regimen that will fit your schedule without causing injury. You can contact me personally at my website www.getfitwithkimtoday.com if you would like to work with me.

## KIDS AND EXERCISE

When I was growing up, we couldn't wait to go play outside. Whether we spent the day at the swimming pool or rode our bicycles all over town, we were outside doing something physical. Occasionally, there was a rainy day when we went to the movies or stayed inside to play video games and read, but that was seldom in West Texas. Advancing technology provides today's kids a sedentary lifestyle in a world of games, videos, computers, etc. at their fingertips. Getting some kids to use their imaginations and play outside can be a challenge for parents.

To engage sedentary kids in activity, limit TV, gaming, and computer time. Restrict these sedentary activities for after supper to ensure that your kids put physical activity first. Reading and playing games with the entire family are great activities but should not replace physical exercise.

Generally, kids have spent all day at school sitting, focusing, and using their brains with little to no physical activity. I highly recommend encouraging your kiddos to run and play, if they are not in any sports *immediately after* school, *before* starting their homework. The excess energy burned helps them to sit still and study. The oxygen-rich blood from exercise feeds their brains helping them focus and better grasp information. Try it and see if their homework doesn't go smoother and quicker!

**For the kids who are actively participating in sports, parents may need to take the opposite approach.** Some kids compete in *several* overlapping sports during the school year. With the ever-growing competitive nature to be the best in their sport, parents may feel their kids must use school breaks to practice or get private lessons to gain an edge over their peers. Unfortunately, this intensity can cause burnout and overtraining, which leads to injury for the young athlete.

**On the flip side:** Encouraging young athletes to try different sports during summer break will teach them new skills, keep them active and social while meeting new people, provide cross training to their main sport, reducing risk of overuse injuries, prevent boredom, and avoid burnout. This allows young athletes the physical and mental break needed from their main sport. They also learn to get out of their comfort zone and possibly find a new talent or interest.

For both the sedentary and competitive kids, summer break is a great time to introduce new activities to your child that they may not otherwise have time to try during the school year. Because the time frame (season) is shorter in the summer, they have an opportunity to try several different activities. From organized sport camps, swimming, martial arts classes, to the arts: painting, photography, and music; there are summer programs offered everywhere. Contact local schools, museums, churches, the YMCA, Boys & Girls Clubs for information on different programs offered near you.

Whether the activities are organized, neighborhood games, or days spent at the swimming pool, the most important thing is that your kids enjoy the activities. When **equating exercise with fun,** we will instill the habit of being physically active, every day, at a young age. They will be more likely to carry a healthy lifestyle on into adulthood. Isn't that really the goal?

**The MOST IMPORTANT FACTOR in getting sedentary children active is to set a good example YOURSELF.** Children are watching *everything* you do. Their interests and habits are typically a reflection of their parents'. If you are constantly complaining about exercise or putting it off, your children will not see the importance of health or look forward to exercise, either. [12]

Lead by example. Exercising – or "playing," as I like to refer to it – is just one more way to connect with and teach your kiddos healthy habits.

---

12   It's easier to prevent bad habits than to break them. – Benjamin Franklin

# IT'S TIME TO PLAY!

Remember when we were kids and our parents had to bribe us to come inside and eat supper? My brother and I could hear my dad whistling two blocks away for us to come home. Nobody had to *make* us "play." It seems the tables turn as we age. We love nap time and dread exercise. All too often, we see people retire, sit in front of the TV for the first time in their lives, and begin to deteriorate – physically and mentally. When you STOP moving, your body loses the ABILITY to move.

**It's time we start "playing" again.**[13]

I categorize people into one of two groups when it comes to exercise; those who **GET** to exercise, and those who **HAVE** to exercise.

## For those who HAVE to exercise:

I challenge you to think back to what you enjoyed doing as a child. Did you participate in a sport, ride your bike all weekend with friends, or play with your pets? Return to those activities, and I promise you will enjoy "playtime" (exercise). Join an intramural sports team, go rollerblading, bike riding, train for a triathlon, swim, or golf. If you are physically unable to play your favorite sport anymore, hire a certified personal trainer who can structure workouts simulating your favorite sports or activities. You will be monitored by them while enjoying the workout.

Be part of a group: Join a local running group. If running is not your idea of a good time, then join a bicycling club or aerobics

13   The world is your playground. – Kim Clinkenbeard

classes. Finding others who enjoy the same activities as you will help you stick with your exercise program.

## For those who GET to exercise:

As an adult, I have spent hours and hours in the gym, not only exercising, but also working. After more than 25 years in the gym, I'm just plain bored! I think this is an issue for many of us who have been exercising for decades. We get bored.

**If our minds are bored, our bodies will suffer.**

The human body needs variety to thrive. Our muscles condition to the same workouts and movements very quickly. This is why you get sore after doing something you haven't done before or in a long time, like heavy yard work, building a tree house for the kids, or going hiking.

When I was in college, I painted the local schools every summer with a crew of other college kids. It was a fun way to make money at a summer job. I remember the first week we were all sore from painting, carrying 5-gallon buckets of paint, and going up and down the ladder 1000 times a day. After the first week, though, the soreness went away because our muscles got used to the movements. Yes, it was physical labor all day, every day, but we no longer got sore from it. My point is, you need to change up your exercise routine; not only for your muscles to continue getting stronger and improve, but so you don't also get bored and stop exercising all together. Keep workouts fresh and fun to ensure good results and that exercise stays on your schedule.

**Here are a few NEW activities I have recently added to change things up and stay motivated.**

- ➢ **LONG BOARD:** It's like a skate board but quite a bit longer and somewhat wider than a regular skateboard. I don't know about you, but falling on the hard asphalt or concrete is not enticing to me - at all. In fact, one of my main goals is to avoid falling at all cost. However, the long board makes it MUCH easier!

    - ◦ Long boarding itself is an awesome core workout! It works on stability, balance, proprioception, agility, and some leg strength to keep it going.

    - ◦ You're outside in the fresh air and sunshine, boosting your mood and vitamin D levels.

    - ◦ There are many other exercises you can do using the long board besides just riding it down the street, like abs, hamstring curls, lunges and wall squats. I incorporate the long board into my clients' workouts for fun.

- ➢ **SPEED BAG:** I grew up watching the *ROCKY* movies (and yes, "crushing" a little on Rocky, himself). Being the forever tom-boy, I have always wanted to learn to hit the speed bag. So, I asked for a speed bag for Christmas one year. I highly recommend it! It's one of my favorite workouts ever.

    - ◦ You get an awesome arm and shoulder workout!

    - ◦ You can work out your stress/frustrations and exercise your body at the same time. I love how exercise provides a positive outlet for stress. I have worked through many life struggles during a workout. (Picture whomever you want on the speed bag while you hit it, and no one will be the wiser. Ha!)

- ◦ It improves hand-eye coordination, timing, speed, focus, and works on your abdominals and core strength.

- ◦ It's easy to incorporate into other exercises. I will hit the speed bag after running or biking to get some upper body work or include it in a circuit workout.

➢ **FRISBEE:** I have never been able to throw a Frisbee well, but now they have a variety of *new* Frisbees that are super easy to throw and catch. The best part? They are CHEAP! Around $8.

- ◦ Throwing a Frisbee is a great way to get your cardio done and have fun at the same time. Not to mention, you may get more of a workout if you have to climb a tree, on top of the house, or swim to the bottom of the pool to get it.

- ◦ It's social! When my husband and I have a lazy Sunday afternoon, we grab the dogs and a couple friends and go throw the Frisbee. It's a great way to tap into your inner child.

- ◦ Again, you are outside getting all the benefits that nature provides us.

➢ **JUST GET OUTSIDE AND PLAY!** It's not rocket science.

- ◦ Chase your kids around in the back yard in a fun game of Tag.

- ◦ Add water balloons to the game in the summer. It's a fun way to cool off and be active.

- If you don't have kids, your dogs will be more than happy to play Tag with you - indoors or outdoors.

- Toss the football or baseball around.

- Start a neighborhood pick-up game of basketball or street hockey.

- Start a walking group in your neighborhood. Meet a few evenings after supper. You can encourage kids to come along on their bikes. You will be inspiring health within your own community, as well as your family.

No matter which category you fall under – the *HAVE to's* OR the *GET to's*- I promise you can find some form of activity you will look forward to doing.

## WHAT YOU NEED TO KNOW ABOUT H.I.I.T. WORKOUTS

As I watched my dog play at the park with some kids the other day, I noticed a correlation to the way I train myself and my clients –

*my basic, fundamental training philosophy:* **H.I.I.T. it hard!**

Dogs and kids are the quintessential examples of INTERVAL TRAINING. If you ever take a moment to watch them play, you will notice they go full speed as hard as they can and then suddenly stop for a break. Whether it's their short attention spans or the fact their little hearts, lungs and bodies need a short recess from the all-out, mach-10 speed, this is the basic principal behind H.I.I.T. work outs.

In my opinion, H.I.I.T. workouts are the absolute **best way to exercise for FAT LOSS** and **Overall Conditioning** and should be incorporated into EVERY exercise program. H.I.I.T. is also something for athletes to consider when trying to gain speed in any sport.

H.I.I.T. stands for *High Intensity Interval Training*, which breaks down into bursts of *INTENSE* workout sessions immediately followed by SHORT periods of *complete rest* OR "active rest." ("Active rest" is classified as anything other than standing still: marching in place, for example.) Workouts can be structured in endless variations incorporating free weights, machines, or only your body weight. H.I.I.T. workouts can also be used in your cardio training. Runners typically categorized this type of workout as a *tempo run* or a *fartlek run*. The rest periods can range from standing still to easy jogging. The possibilities are endless and determined by your individual fitness level, goals, and sport.

This is not to say that endurance activities at a moderate pace don't have their place. Remember the classic tale of the tortoise and the hare? Steady wins the race, and building a strong cardio-respiratory base (for endurance) is *crucial* in racing and in life functions. It takes a lot of endurance to chase the dog (or the kids) around the park when they steal the Frisbee!

If you are short on time or just want to spice things up a bit, H.I.I.T. workouts are something to add to your routine. However, you should *never* structure an exercise program consisting *only* of H.I.I.T. workouts. Incorporating 1-3 sessions of H.I.I.T. workouts per week is plenty without risking injury.

# HOW DO YOU GET STARTED WITH AN EXERCISE ROUTINE?

First Things First:

> Set a regular bed time and wake time.

> Get a physical from your physician that includes a full blood panel, testing everything, including the sex hormones (estrogen, testosterone, progesterone) and thyroid (T3, T4). Ask for a copy for your personal records. This may be your saving grace at some point.

> Take the recommended Rx medications/supplements as directed by your doctor.

> Set a regular bed time and wake time. Oh, did I say that already? It must be important!

> Schedule your workout. If exercise is not scheduled, it typically will not get done, even with the best intensions.

  ◦ Set specific days AND a specific time to exercise.

  ◦ Put your workout on your calendar as a *meeting*.

  ◦ DO NOT reschedule your workout.

> Prepare and plan ahead.

  ◦ Make sure you have your workout clothes, shoes, water etc. with you. Especially if you intend to leave for the gym straight from work or school.

> Set yourself up for success.

  ◦ If you cannot feasibly exercise two hours a day, six days a week, then don't make that schedule for yourself.

- ○ Pick an activity you enjoy doing and will look forward to each day.

- ○ Get a workout partner or a trainer. *Accountability is key to long term success in an exercise program, especially if you are just starting.*

➤ Be consistent and persistent.[14]

- ○ **Consistency is the single most important factor of being successful.**

  The most successful people *consistently* work at whatever it is they want to accomplish even when they don't *feel* like it - whether it's exercise, eating right, studying, saving money, or following through with commitments. [15]

➤ Learn how to set goals.

- ○ Have a plan to reach those goals.

➤ Incorporate exercise throughout your day, if you don't have time to designate 30 minutes straight to exercise.

➤ Understand that you will NEVER lose weight by exercise alone. You cannot out-exercise a bad diet.

➤ View exercise as the means to stay physically fit and active, so you can live the lifestyle you want to live, for as long as you live.

---

14   Don't give up! The beginning is always the hardest. -Unknown

15   Success cannot be bought, it can only be rented. And rent is due every day. -Unknown

*P.S.*

*Don't put limitations on yourself like: "I'll never be able to keep up in such-and-such class/group because I'm too out-of-shape." Or "I'm too old to run a marathon." Or whatever your "limiting self-talk" is. I have done many triathlons (including 70.3 Ironman Triathlons) with people who were pregnant (noticeably pregnant!), who had no legs (they did the entire race with their arms!), and who were the young age of 90! There is always the possibility of achieving your dreams. Sometimes, we just need to get out of our own way.*

DREAM BIG FRIENDS!!

# REST and RECOVERY

# The MOST IMPORTANT components of any exercise and nutrition program are REST and RECOVERY.

They are also the *LEAST utilized and incorporated components* used to enhance quality of life and performance. It's important to understand that REST and RECOVERY are two *different* things.

> **REST** is the time spent sleeping as well as the time spent *not* exercising. How you spend the "free" time is very important to how your body heals from strenuous activity like exercise and sports.

> **RECOVERY** refers to the *techniques* and *strategies* you use to help maximize your body's ability to heal and repair as well as the time spent standing versus sitting versus lying down.

Rest and Recovery are multifaceted. They are when you recharge your batteries: brain function and memory, nervous system repair, muscle repair, digestion, chemical and hormone balance, mental and emotional states, etc. Of all these different systems (Neurological, Hormonal, and Structural) requiring Recovery, the Structural System is where we put most of our effort. This includes muscles, tendons, ligaments, and bones.

While the Structural System recovery is important, the Neuro-logical and Hormonal aspects are equally important to overall health and quality of life. Becoming too focused on one system over the others encourages your health to eventually suffer, as all three are interrelated.

**Finding a balance of REST and RECOVERY along with proper diet and exercise should be the goal of EVERY fitness program.** While I believe, "your workouts should *support* your lifestyle," I do *NOT* believe your fitness program should *be your life*. It should not take over your life, restrict your lifestyle, keep you from friends and family, or leave you feeling lonely or exhausted. Incorporate what you can and what you feel is most important to your overall health goals. Leave the rest behind.

*A happy and healthy person performs better and has the time and energy for others.*

**There are many tools that help you RECOVER** from illness, strenuous activity, sports, exercise, stress, etc. They include:

1) Hydration
2) Nutrition
3) Massage
4) Steam room
5) Epsom salt bath
6) SMR (Self-Myofascial Release) – foam rolling
7) ART (Active Release Technique) or Rossiter – trigger point release
8) Yoga or Stretching
9) Compression
10) Heat/Ice
11) Stress management

I have implemented and recommend to my clients all the above techniques at one time or another. They all have their place and effectiveness. I have outlined strategies to help you implement most of these forms of recovery into your lifestyle throughout this book. With a little guidance and trial and error, you will find what works best for you.

## STRESS MANAGEMENT[16]

Quickly rate your stress level on a scale from 1 to 10 with 10 being "I think my head might explode I'm so stressed!" Now, make a mental list of the health issues you are currently dealing with, like obesity, high blood pressure, thyroid disorders, headaches, irritability etc. Notice the correlation between your level of stress and the degree of the health issues you listed. High levels of chronic stress are linked to the major diseases plaguing our nation: cancer, heart disease, high blood pressure, obesity, diabetes, and more.

So......

*What constitutes stress?*
*What about the "good" stresses in life?*
*Do they lead to disease, too?*

### There are two types of stress: ACUTE and CHRONIC.

**ACUTE stress** can be something good, like planning a wedding, moving, starting a new job, starting an exercise program, or learning a new skill. These are all situations which usually start immediately and have an end or deadline. They may be good

---

16   "I read this article that said the typical symptoms of stress are eating too much, impulse buying, and driving too fast. Are they kidding? That's my idea of a perfect day!" - Someecards

things like those listed above or bad things like catching the flu, road rage, or breaking your leg.

ACUTE stress is temporary, and your body can handle and quickly recover from this type of stress without long-term damage.

## MY STORY

*A true story of an acutely stressful day in the life of "me":*

I lost my wallet.

Yes, I was multi-tasking, running errands and trying to get EVERYTHING done that I had put off until the last possible minute. The bad thing was, I had been so distracted by all my "duties" as a -------------------- (fill in the blank) to whomever in my life, that I didn't even realize I had lost it, until the *next day* when I needed to pay the swimming pool fee. Luckily, they let me swim anyway. I figured, why worry about the wallet now? It couldn't get much worse in an hour if someone *had* stolen my identity. I wished them better luck with being me than I've had - wink, wink - and went about my swim workout.

When I got home, one would think the first thing I would do was go on a mad hunt to find my missing life (a.k.a. wallet). Nope! Not this girl. Distraction grabbed hold of me with its nasty hand again. I began paperwork, emails, and bill paying. This was the one and only time I have EVER been thankful to pay bills. I couldn't do it because—you guessed it—NO WALLET! That's when I gave myself the "Hello McFly" head slap. (If you don't know the movie reference, it's *Back to the Future*. I'm showing my age here, but it's a great 80's flick if you haven't seen it.) I finally went on the anxiety stricken mad hunt for my wallet; finally finding it after a two-hour search of every crack and crevasse, including the grocery baskets at HEB. As I took a break from the search by raiding the fridge, I caught a glimpse of its little leather case. Yes, it was in the fridge. What a relief! Not only was the anxiety-ridden food binge averted, but I didn't have to try and figure out who and where to call to cancel myself and start a fresh identity.

## HOW TO MANAGE ACUTE STRESS

Losing my wallet made me wonder: do grown-ups need **ADULT TIME-OUTS?** Not for doing something bad, necessarily. Well, ok. Some of us need time-outs for that too – a.k.a. prison. Adults do need time-outs, so we can get our heads on straight, refocus our thoughts, and keep up with the important things in life, like *where did I leave little Johnny*? As daily life and business stress piles on, I don't really "listen" to my husband, family, friends, etc. My true attention is elsewhere. This also means that I'm not listening to myself, either. (Especially since we all tend to put ourselves last on the list.)

Here are some of my ADULT TIME-OUT favorites:

➤ Schedule **QUIET TIME**. Taking 10-20 minutes every day to read my Bible and/or a daily devotional, pray, listen to a Christian podcast or music, help me relax and keep my stress levels in check. My perspective is refreshed. When my priorities are in order, my ability to handle stress is much better because I know where my focus is – on God and not myself and crazy to-do list.

➤ **EXERCISE** is another way to regroup every day and get my focus back. It happens that exercise also doubles as a way to burn off calories, get in physical shape, and make us look and feel better. Try 20-30 minutes of exercise. It works for me. (I'm not in prison yet. Ha!)

➤ **LAUGH OUT LOUD!** Laughter relaxes blood vessels and increases blood flow -- the exact opposite of what your blood vessels do when you are stressed. Worry has never added one day to anybody's life or solved one problem. I encourage you to find the humor in stressful situations. Surround yourself with people who encourage you, lift your spirits, and make you LAUGH!

> **"Laughter is the best medicine."** I believe this is true, and there is scientific evidence to support that statement. Studies have shown that laughter helps the pituitary gland release its own pain-suppressing opiates to help you feel better and get pain-free sleep. WHAT?! I'm in!

Laughter has also been proven to:

- ◦ Lower blood pressure
- ◦ Increase vascular blood flow and oxygenation of the blood
- ◦ Give a workout to the diaphragm and abdominal, respiratory, facial, leg, and back muscles, helping you to feel more relaxed afterwards
- ◦ Reduce certain stress hormones, such as cortisol and adrenaline

- ○ Increase the response of tumor and disease-killing cells, such as Gamma-interferon and T-cells, boosting your immunity

- ○ Defend against respiratory infections –even reducing the frequency of colds– by immunoglobulin in saliva

- ○ Improve alertness, creativity, learning ability, and memory

It can be to find humor in stressful situations. I like to describe myself as a Type B personality trapped in a Type A+++ body, but it's worth a try if you can add years to your life. Happy years at that.

➢ **LOVE** - Of course we think of our spouses, families, and even our pets, but random acts of kindness and volunteering can spark heart-healthy feelings of satisfaction, gratitude and self-worth. Research indicates those who volunteer have lower rates of heart disease, live longer, and are overall more physically and mentally fit.

You don't have to ADD another thing on your to-do list. Make loving others and volunteering simple by:

- ○ Offering to walk your neighbor's dog while walking your own puppy.

- ○ Complimenting a stranger in line at the grocery store. I know you've done this too, thought to yourself, "she looks really pretty in that color" but didn't tell them. I decided that every time I complimented someone (stranger or not) in my mind, I would TELL them! You will be amazed at how a simple compliment can brighten someone's face and make you feel good and "brighter," too!

- ◦ It doesn't have to take money or even much time. Think outside the box!

➢ **RELAX!** Go see a movie, pop bubble wrap, journal, take a stroll in the park, or just relax in a bubble bath with a good book. Try to do something every day for at least 15 minutes that makes you relax.

Make time for a much-needed ADULT TIME-OUT. By finding something that slows you down for a few minutes daily, you can be the best YOU for everyone in your life.

Problems occur when **ACUTE stress** turns into **CHRONIC stress.** Chronic stress can make you sick and cause underlying health conditions to surface.

**CHRONIC stress** typically results from a negative life event, comes on gradually, wears you down, and seems like it may never end. This can include losing your job, learning to live with an incurable disease, working an unsatisfying job, dealing with difficult people, or maybe just not being able to cope with life in general.

**When managing stress is not an ongoing way of life, your body will suffer the consequences and begin to rebel.**

This leads to a domino effect.... lack of sleep.... fatigue.... poor judgment.... no exercise.... poor diet.... moodiness.... forgetfulness.... troubled relationships.... poor work performance.... depression.... weight gain.... and finally, diseases such as heart disease, diabetes, cancer, thyroid disease, etc.

Now, go back and look at the list you made earlier. Did lack of sleep make the top of your list? I have noticed with myself and clients that...

*the first thing to suffer at the hands of stress is SLEEP.*

It begins with not being able to "turn your mind off." We try to get by on less and less, putting sleep at the end of our priority list. The first thing we cut back when we need more time is NOT the TV, but SLEEP. *Left unchecked, lack of sleep is the doorway to all the other issues mentioned above* (and close to being in that order). I believe that lack of sleep could also be called the *Silent Killer*.

When faced with high levels of acute or chronic stress, make a good night's sleep your #1 PRIORITY, and you will be more successful at managing your stress, overcoming it, and fighting off life threatening disease!

You can use all or some of the above forms of Recovery and achieve a degree of success. However, if you are not getting enough sleep, you will never *fully* heal. Sleep is essential to the health and repair of your body.

**SLEEP is the MOST IMPORTANT element in a successful, healthy lifestyle.**

## SLEEP

As kids, we fight it. As adults, we cherish it. In today's fast paced society, it's become a luxury some fear we will never have again.

*Can you remember the last time you woke up feeling well rested and ready to tackle the day?*

If you answered, "No" you are not alone. Insomnia is rapidly becoming an epidemic affecting 1 in 3 U.S. adults, with the majority being women. Lack of sleep is directly related to loss of cognitive skills, depression, lack of energy, weight gain, obesity, and ultimately the diseases related to obesity.

Many things can contribute to sleepless nights:

- Stress
- Prescription and OTC Medications (high blood pressure, thyroid, hormones, allergy and cold medications, pain medications)
- Medical conditions like restless leg syndrome and sleep apnea, depression and anxiety disorders, menopause, thyroid disorders, etc.

Pinpointing some of these can help you and your doctor diagnose possible causes for your insomnia. Once the above mentioned are ruled out as causes of your sleeplessness, it's time to address your HABITS and LIFESTYLE. Even if you do not suffer from chronic insomnia, it's worth taking a closer look at your habits and lifestyle *now, before* you develop any sleep issues. Whatever the culprit for your insomnia, there are things you can change *today* that can help you catch some ZZZ's tonight.

There are several ways to prepare your mind and body for sleep other than the known facts of reducing caffeine, sugar, and alcohol in the late afternoons.

**SIDE BAR:** It's a myth that alcohol promotes sleep. It may help you initially sleep for a few hours, but then you will suddenly find yourself wide awake and unable to fall back to sleep. Alcohol is a very common and recognized CAUSE of insomnia. Similarly, many sleep aids have a "rebound" effect, causing you to wake up with thoughts racing, leaving you unable to fall back to sleep.

**PROPER NUTRITION, HYDRATION, and EXERCISE all contribute to the QUALITY of SLEEP you get – or don't get.**

Here's the scoop:

➢ *WHAT you eat and drink, as well as WHEN you eat and drink, BOTH affect your sleep.*

Going to bed on a **full stomach with hard-to-digest foods** like red meat, cheese, nuts, etc. will lead to disrupted sleep. You can expect to experience at best, discomfort and bloating and at worst, acid reflux. Long term consequences of acid reflux can lead to insomnia and even esophageal cancer.

I recommend **eating your last substantial meal at least 3 hours prior to bedtime** to allow for proper digestion. A small snack like a green smoothie, cucumbers, sauerkraut, or easily digestible fruit will keep you satisfied without interfering with your sleep. The magnesium found in many fruits and vegetables also helps you relax and get better quality sleep. Magnesium - whether through an Epsom salt bath at night, supplements before bed, or topical creams - is proven to help with sleep and constipation.

➤ *DEHYDRATION* is a leading cause of Irritable Bowel Syndrome (IBS) and other digestive issues, restless leg syndrome, headaches, muscle cramps, etc. which all contribute to insomnia. Needless to say, drinking a lot of water before bed can also disrupt sleep.

The solution is to stay hydrated throughout the day especially after exercise. This helps ensure dehydration is not causing your ailments. If it's hard for you to drink enough water throughout the day, try to get some of your hydration through your foods. Soups, smoothies, watery foods (like cucumbers, watermelon, other fruits and veggies), and herbal teas are great ways to stay hydrated in addition to water. Relaxing teas like chamomile and "sleepy time tea" also help you sleep. Peppermint and licorice root teas aid in digestion and keep you hydrated. Just try to drink them about an hour before bed, so you aren't up ten times during the night for a potty break. That's a little counterproductive. As with all "natural" remedies, they may or may not work for you, but it's worth a shot.

> **SIDE BAR:** I like to mix Peppermint, Licorice Root, and "Sleepy" tea together, sometimes adding a slice of orange and a cinnamon stick.

➤ *LACK OF vigorous EXERCISE and PHYSICAL ACTIVITY* throughout the day can actually **CAUSE fatigue** and lead to **sleepless nights**. We should move as much as possible during the day and incorporate at least 30 minutes of vigorous exercise six days a week. Being active metabolizes our food, oxygenates our bodies, and promotes quality, deep sleep. However, note that vigorously exercising within two hours of bedtime can cause a spike in blood pressure and heart rate, as well as dehydration, which in turn will disrupt your sleep.

➤ *Make your BEDROOM a WORK-FREE ZONE.* Don't take your work to bed with you. Set a bedtime and leave your unfinished tasks for tomorrow. This will help you turn your brain "off" to life stresses. Think about it like this; if not fully rested and recharged, you cannot be the best parent, co-worker, boss, spouse, friend, etc. you want to be.

➤ *Reduce or eliminate all AUDIBLE and VISUAL STIMU- LATION.* This includes watching TV or using any other electronic devices in bed. While a good *Seinfeld* re-run may help take your mind off your problems for a moment, the blue light emitted from your TV, phone, and computer can disrupt your circadian rhythm and the production of the sleep hormone, melatonin.

As I lay awake one sleepless night listening to the battle of the bands between my husband and dog, Mazy, I noticed a few things. First, a dog can hold her own in the snoring department. All we needed was a baritone, and we could take our act on the road. GET EARPLUGS if you have this same problem with your spouse or live in an area where you can hear the sounds of the city.

Second, we have several electronic devices putting off just enough light to cast shadows on the walls! So, I put a piece of tape on all the little lights we don't need – the smoke detector, cable box, TV etc. I also got blackout curtains (I put them behind my pretty decorative curtains) since our bedroom windows face a street lamp. Another tip is to cover your alarm clock with a wash cloth or bandana (that's what I use). Besides the unnecessary glow, clock watching causes stress, making it difficult to fall to sleep.

Why do we need *total darkness?* It allows our bodies to produce the hormone, melatonin and regulate our "body clock," known as the circadian rhythm. We cannot sleep without it. Natural light, artificial light, and darkness all affect the production of melatonin by the body (the brain's Pineal Gland). Darkness activates the production of melatonin while light suppresses it. For this reason, it's extremely important to give our bodies proper exposure to light and dark at appropriate times of day. This, along with temperature, also affects our circadian rhythm.

There are other ways to get more melatonin. Foods like bananas and walnuts contain melatonin. If allergic to these foods, another option is Over-The-Counter (OTC) melatonin supplements, available in the vitamin aisle. Be sure to discuss this supplement with your health care provider, as further research is needed to prove the effectiveness of OTC melatonin and improved sleep.

➢ *COLOR IT AMBER.* Amber light helps your eyes and brain *r e l a x.*

Unlike bright light and blue light emitting devices, amber-colored lights will not disrupt the production of melatonin or your circadian rhythm.

If you're like me and enjoy reading a silly book on your e-reader before bed, purchase a pair of amber-colored glasses. They cost about $10 and filter the blue light without having to change your light bulbs. They are also great to wear while working at the computer for long periods of time.

If glasses aren't your thing, there is an app called "f.lux" that reduces blue light emitted from your computer screen. (There may be more apps that do this same thing.) The app can be scheduled to come on when the sun starts to set and to turn off with the sunrise to mimic natural light. This helps reduce eye stress while working at the computer. However, I still highly recommend completing your computer work at least 1-2 hours before bed.

Another effective, and my *favorite* light-filtering tool, is an amber-colored screen protector. This can be used instead of the glasses. These flexible amber-colored screens can be ordered and customized to fit over any device; phone, Kindle, tablet etc. It's put on your device like other screen protectors. I highly recommend this for anyone who likes to read books on their electronic devices before bed.

➢ *Make a RELAXING BEDTIME ROUTINE.* The hour before your bedtime should be reserved for relaxing and preparing for sleep.

Suggestions for setting up your routine:

- ◦ Set a bedtime and wake time and stick to them!

- ◦ Make a list of what you need to do for tomorrow. This way you won't be thinking all night long about what to remember to do in the morning.

- ◦ Prepare your breakfast and what you need to take with you the next day, so you're not rushed or stressed in the morning.

- ◦ THEN RELAX YOUR BODY AND MIND.

- Take a warm shower or Epsom salt bath.

- Drink sleepy tea or other non-caffeinated herbal tea.

- Listen to soft music or read (wearing your amber glasses of course).

➤ *Purchase a SOUND MACHINE.* I bought one for another project but thought, "why not try it in the bedroom?" The best sleep of my life has been on scuba diving trips. So, I picked the *ocean waves* setting. It just so happens that the sound of running water (rain, ocean, river) has been found to have therapeutic effects. It worked for me. Now, even the dogs remind me to turn it on before we go to bed.

➤ *SLEEP WITH A BODY PILLOW.* And no, your bed buddy doesn't count. At the suggestion of my massage therapist, I finally gave it a try after putting it off for a year. I'll admit I'm a little hard headed sometimes, but when you have a husband and a couple of dogs (or in your case maybe a kid) sleeping with you, it's difficult to add a body pillow, too! What can I say? Pain motivates.

As a side sleeper, my hips and shoulder would constantly get out of alignment. Eventually the pain would disrupt my sleep. After adding the pillow between my legs and arms, my hips stayed aligned, and my shoulder stopped hurting. Now I sleep with it when I'm extremely active and in heavy training which, for me, leads to misalignments. If pain frequently wakes you up, this may be a solution.

➤ *CHECK THE TEMPERATURE.* Research indicates the **ideal temperature for restful sleep is 66° - 68°F**. A mild drop in body temperature helps induce sleep. But if the room becomes *uncomfortably* hot or cold, you are more likely to wake up. Try adjusting your thermostat for a few days to find the perfect temperature where you get the most sleep.

> *TRACK IT.* If you are unsure about the quality of your sleep habits or question if you're getting enough deep sleep, then investigate the phone apps and fitness trackers designed to track your sleep. My favorite fitness tracker tells me how long it took me to fall asleep, how many hours of light and deep sleep I got, how many times I woke up during the night, and more. It's worth the small investment to identify your sleep habits.

NOTE: While I'm not comfortable endorsing specific brands in this book because companies go out-of-business and science/technology advances, I am happy to guide and share with you my favorite brand names if you contact me directly through my website at www.getfitwithkimtoday.com.

I'm always chasing a better night's SLEEP, especially if it doesn't involve taking medications. I have incorporated all these suggestions for better sleep, and they really do work! However, this has not always been the case for me. I did go through time when my doctor "made" me take a prescription sleep aid.

## MY STORY

In the FITNESS section, I shared with you some of the issues that led to my diagnosis of thyroid disorder and Premature Ovarian Failure. A primary symptom was *INSOMNIA*. For about three months, I did not sleep more than two hours a night. My body was shutting down from lack of hormones and sleep. I had reached the point where I was not able to sleep without the aid of a prescription sleeping pill. I say the doctor "made" me take it because I am a "naturalist" – someone who treats and heals their body with food instead of medication. Thanks to that doctor and my husband for explaining that I needed a prescription to help me get back on a sleep cycle allowing my body to heal. While my motives were good, I was not allowing myself to get well unless I swallowed my pride along with the medication. This was a journey in and of itself. Taking the prescription sleep aid for about three months helped regulate my body clock until I could sleep for eight hours on my own. I will testify that IT SAVED ME!

The short-term use of a prescription sleep aid has its purpose. I suggest formulating a plan with your doctor on how to take it and for how long. I was able to take a small dose for a short time with little to no side effects and have not needed a prescription sleep aid since. I can sleep using the strategies outlined in this chapter. However, if there comes a time when prescription help is needed again, I will not hesitate to work with my doctor to find the best treatment.

Getting and staying asleep can be an art-form. We can even get to the point where we must resort to prescription sleep aids. Chemical aids do serve a purpose in their need to help people over an initial obstacle to regain their health. Unfortunately for many, their bodies come to rely on the medication completely and suffer from intense side-effects. This was not the case for me, but it was for a good friend of mine.

After suffering a heart attack, a he was prescribed a sleeping pill to help him relax and get the necessary rest he needed for recovery. He began feeling the side effects of the sleeping pills in a very drastic way. It was more than slight dizziness for him. He felt like somebody spiked the punch with tequila; spinning ceiling fans and all. He was totally knocked out for 8 hours (even with a reduced dosage) and had no recollection of eating, doing laundry or having conversations with his wife in the middle of the night. The effects of the sleeping pill would stay with him well into the morning after waking up.

We had two very different experiences with prescription sleep aids. My point here is that *everybody is different.* Sometimes short-term, specific use of a sleep aid can be a tool used to help you get the vital sleep your body needs to heal. As a patient, *you must be your own advocate.* If something isn't working, speak up and tell your doctor. (Find a doctor who *listens* to you!) Knowing what works for you is great, but sometimes knowing what *does not* work is even *more helpful* in conquering insomnia.

Before trying temporary solutions like OTC or prescription sleep aids, try incorporating some or all the techniques and gadgets listed in this section. They are not expensive or hard to find. In the long run, it will be a healthier option for your body and benefit your sleep long term.

# FOOD

# FOOD is the most abused "drug" and the hardest to overcome.[17]

Let me clarify why I made such a strong statement.

I have never struggled with anything that is recognized as an addiction – drugs, alcohol, gambling, shopping, or even cigarettes, just to name a few. I cannot even guess what those struggles are like or understand how hard it is to overcome them. What I can relate to is struggling with *FOOD ADDICTION.*

I don't mean to belittle anyone's struggle with addiction. Please know I am coming from a place of compassion and love for you and your efforts to heal from those addictions. However, I must say that food, to me, *is the most difficult "drug" to overcome because* it is something that we literally *CANNOT LIVE WITHOUT.* We can't avoid it. It's always around us. We must continually buy it, store it, cook it, be around it, think about it, and put it in our bodies. As hard as it is to not think about alcohol for an alcoholic, it's *impossible* to not think about food for *everyone.* The kicker is that this "drug" we call FOOD is everywhere, easily accessible, and legal!

The food "drug" even has its own "pushers" and "dealers." Usually, these "pushers" and "dealers" are our friends, family, co-workers – those closest to us. The very people who you hope would be on your side *helping* you overcome your food addiction may consciously or subconsciously sabotage your effort to "kick the habit."

People struggling with food feel the same emotions and think

---

17    1 Corinthians 6:13 "You say, 'Food for the stomach and the stomach for food, and God will destroy them both.'"

the same thoughts as those struggling with other addictions. The guilt, shame, embarrassment, defeat, failure, and (for some) self-hate is very real.

The social stigma associated with FOOD ADDICTION can be harsher for those struggling with this type of addiction. Overweight people are viewed as lazy, weak, unmotivated, and flippant regarding their health. While those who are under-weight are viewed as being too disciplined, vain, selfish, and having the wrong priorities.

## MY STORY

My struggle with food began at the end of my senior year in high school after I made collegiate twirler. It was required that I lose 30 lbs. to be eligible to twirl at the football games. I weighed 120 lbs. at the time. Ironically, I have never been viewed as overweight. Losing that amount of weight was impossible, and I ended up quitting the line. That left a shameful and self-destructive pattern of dieting throughout much of my life.

My quest for the perfect weight loss diet and desire to be "skinny" was disguised as motivation for eating healthy and being fit for "my health" for many years. This experience led me to find my passion for and career in fitness and nutrition.

Little did I know, however, that God would use my drive for perfection (and later my injuries and illnesses, also) to teach me about nutrition, exercise, fitness, health, myself, others, and Him! Whatever my motivations were, I was passionate about finding answers for myself and others. When you're passionate about something, studying is easy.

Since 1991, I have diligently studied, researched, and obtained national certifications in Nutrition, Exercise, and Functional Medicine (and many sub categories of each).

What I learned about "diets" and fanatical exercise programs is that eventually, *they all fail.* I couldn't maintain any "diet" or the results long term. No matter how "fit" I got or how "perfect" I looked, I was still never happy with ME. By dieting, I was only setting myself up for failure after failure because none of them had longevity. Continuously failing at something will eventually leave you defeated. ***The cool thing was once I completely gave up on the idea of "perfection," all the stress and pressure left along with the unwanted pounds.***

## When I began to see my HEALTH as worth the effort, *then the effort had worth.*[18]

Understand, I still make a conscience decision *every single day* to exercise and to eat foods that are good for my body (and skip the candy). There are times I'm successful and times I'm not. It's a daily choice[19] – sometimes minute by minute - just like it's a choice to not chase down the guy that nearly ran you off the

---

18  Learn to be more thankful for what you are than guilty for what you are not. Cut the threads of guilt with Grace. – Lysa Terkeurst

19  1 Corinthians 10:23 "'I have the right to do anything,' you say – but not everything is beneficial. 'I have the right to do anything' – but not everything is constructive."

road with an equal level of road rage; just like it's a choice to be grateful or find the good in situations; just like it's a choice to go to work instead of sleeping late. Sometimes learning what NOT to do is most important. Ultimately, like me, *YOU are in control of your choices.*

This passion for nutrition and fitness along with my overwhelming desire to help others find healthy choices for themselves still drives me to learn and share. The difference now is that my passions for God and helping others are much stronger than anything else. [20]

**TIP:**     *Stop trying to be perfect.*
          *Strive to be better than you were.*

We all mess up and fall off the wagon in all areas that we are trying to change. Of course, we tend to beat ourselves up when this happens. We focus so hard on trying to be "good" (or worse, "perfect") when we should instead be focusing on *IMPROVING.*

**Perfection is our enemy!** We all know that's a lost cause, and we will NEVER get there!

Why strive and put all your efforts into something that's impossible to attain? For me, striving for perfection leads to PRIDE. I find myself putting more importance on Myself, My goals, My problems, My success than on God and His will for me. When pride creeps in, I feel like *the harder I work, the worse I get and the further away my faith and goals seem.*[1] Thankfully, God humbles me so I'm forced to set perfection and pride aside and re-focus. I must *CHOOSE*

20   1 Corinthians 10:31 "So whether you eat or drink or whatever you do, do it all for the glory of God."

to let perfection and pride go.

In choosing to *focus on improving* instead, the stress leaves, and we will be re-energized in body, mind and spirit - becoming self-LESS. God doesn't expect us to be perfect, just obedient.

Read that again: *God doesn't expect us to be PERFECT, just OBEDIENT.*

What a relief!!

If God doesn't expect perfection, why should we? This applies to our expectations of others as well. Let's give ourselves and others a break. Do what we are supposed to do each day, and ask for help when we can't (God may send you help from others you would never have thought to ask). Perfection is boring anyway! Some of my favorite things about the people in my life are their imperfections. [1] I'd rather be flawed than boring any day!

*"To all perfection I see a limit, but your commands are boundless." Psalm 119:960*

I made the bold statement that *food is an issue for everyone.* Here's one reason why.

- In the U.S., 68.5% of adults are overweight (that's more than 2/3 the adult population).

- 34.9% of those adults are obese.

- 31.8% of children and adolescents (ages 2-19) are overweight.

- 16.9% of those children (ages 2-19) are obese.

*The kicker? This was data from 2011-2012. The numbers continue to rise every year!*

- WORLDWIDE in 2014, *more than* 1.9 billion adults, 18 years and older, were overweight. Of these over 600 million were obese.

- Overall, about 13% of the WORLD's adult population (11% of men and 15% of women) was obese in 2014.

Those are shocking statistics.[21] And to think, these numbers are from two or more years ago. Food Addiction – overeating - is recognizably an issue worldwide. [22]

The abuse of food and the emotional connections to food are understood by ALL. (The emotional and spiritual aspects to any addiction must be addressed before healing can occur. We will dive into that later in the FAITH section.) We can all relate to situations when our eating habits have not been stellar. Maybe it lasted a week, and maybe it has been going on for years. Some of us hide our struggles better than others.

## *It's time to take responsibility for our actions and our health.*

FOOD IS THE PLACE WE CAN START MAKING SIGNIFICANT CHANGES IN OUR HEALTH - EVEN IF WE ARE PHYSICALLY OR EMOTIONALLY CHALLENGED.

In the quest for health – no matter your motivation - there is confusion in what to eat. Science has proven that certain foods

---

21   "More die in the United States of too much food than too little." – John Kenneth Galbraith

22   "We are all in the same boat. You might as well grab a paddle." – Kim Clinkenbeard

release "feel good" chemicals in our brains while other foods cause us to feel hyper or agitated. Some foods make us feel energized and focused while others make us sleepy and relaxed. There is no argument that food directly affects our energy level and mood. Food is powerful stuff. Some argue food is just as powerful as chemical drugs. I agree.

Like medicine and drugs, the power of food to heal you or kill you is very real.[23] The question is....

## WHAT IS FOOD?

Simply stated: (from a nutrition standpoint) FOOD IS ENERGY - *fuel for your body*.

> **SIDE BAR:** I am not going to go into great scientific detail about food, calories, or exactly how food and nutrition work in the body. For purposes of this book, I will keep the explanations very simplified and general.

The BASICS:

- FOOD contains:
  - *Macro-nutrients* which are carbohydrates, fats, and proteins
  - *Micro-nutrients* which are vitamins and minerals
  - *Fiber* – both soluble and insoluble
  - Water

---

23    "Let food be thy medicine and medicine be thy food." – Hippocrates, 460 B.C.

- Micro-nutrients, fiber, and water are found in Macro-nutrients.

- FOOD (Energy) is commonly measured in calories.

- Carbohydrates have 4 calories per one gram.

- Proteins have 4 calories per one gram.

- Fats contain 9 calories per one gram.

- Alcohol contains 7-14 calories per one gram.

**NOTE:** *Alcohol is not considered a food because we can live without it. It's important to include it for those who drink. I want you to be aware of the how nutrient-deficient alcohol contributes to weight gain.*

All the above, except for alcohol, are necessary for health and survival, but not all are found in every food source. Therefore, it's crucial to eat a well-balanced diet containing carbohydrates, fats, and proteins.

It's important to understand the fundamentals of food and nutrition to help you determine what a *well-balanced diet* is. This knowledge *will save you a lot of time, frustration, money, and help you recognize fad diet schemes.*

When you're sick, tired, or frustrated and just want solutions, the last thing you need is a scientific dissertation on nutrition. So, I will barely scratch the surface of basic nutrition here. This will help you find your nutrition profile (not a short term "diet") that you can live with for the rest of your life. I'm here to teach you how to dissect the "quick fix diets" and never get duped by fancy marketing, again.

Understanding the basics of nutrition is the first step.

It will help you find the answers to some big questions like:

1) Should I be a vegetarian?
2) Why low-carb, high-protein diets never work long term.
3) Why "bullet proof coffee" and other high oil-concentrated diets wreak havoc on your body.
4) Which foods heal, and which foods kill?
5) What should we be eating?
6) What is moderation, and can we even do it?

## WHAT, WHY, HOW MUCH

**PROTEIN:** Protein is necessary for *every* function of the body because it's in *every* cell of the body.

Protein is necessary for proper muscle contraction, health, and repair of our muscles, bones, and skin. Protein is made up of amino acids and provides some energy. The heart is a muscle and therefore needs adequate protein to function properly. Tendons and ligaments require protein to stay strong, pliable, and repair properly.

Protein is found in meats, poultry, fish, eggs, dairy, vegetables, nuts, beans, legumes, and grains.

Protein in meats is a COMPLETE Protein. Complete proteins contain ALL the amino acids a body cannot make on its own. Most plant proteins are INCOMPLETE. *This is why a strictly vegetarian diet is not typically adequate for good overall health.* You must eat a VERY *wide variety* of plants *daily* to supply the body's need for protein. Let's face it - most of us *will not do this.*

It takes A LOT of preparation and determination to be a healthy, successful vegetarian. (And in my opinion, a happy one.)

Because the body does not store protein the way it stores fats and carbohydrates, it's necessary to eat protein DAILY. How much protein you need is based on your age, sex, health, and level of physical activity.

*TOO MUCH Protein in the diet equals* high ketosis and stress on the kidneys contributing to kidney stones and nutrient deficiencies—since protein has little vitamins and minerals—and constipation, due to the lack of fiber, as well as the drying nature of protein. It takes a lot of water to digest protein and move it through the digestive track.

ULTIMATELY, *you will SUFFER from constipation, low energy, brain fog, and eventually, weight gain, because you will not be getting enough fiber, vitamins and minerals in your diet if you eat a very high protein diet.*

**When not getting enough nutrients, your body continues to send hunger signals that cannot be ignored until you give it those nutrients.** At first, a high protein diet will have an appetite suppressing effect, because protein is very satiating, but that will soon end.

*NOT ENOUGH Protein in your diet* and your muscles, tendons, and ligaments cannot grow, heal, or repair properly. You will not get adequate vitamin B-12 (among other things) as it's only found in meat. Vitamin B-12 helps with fat and sugar metabolism. Not enough vitamin B-12 leads to low energy and weakened immunity. Because protein acts as a buffer, not eating enough protein will leave your body in an acidic state which can cause a host of health issues leading to obesity and disease.

> **NOTE:** Eating too much highly processed foods and fast foods also leaves the body in an acidic state.

**FAT:** Fats supply 60% of the body's RESTING ENERGY.

Fat is responsible for the body's absorption of four key vitamins (A, D, E, K). Fat helps keep joints and the digestive tract (bowels) lubed and working properly, and fat plays an important role in cholesterol levels.

Fat is found in meats, nuts, oils, butter, eggs, avocadoes, olives, fish....

*TOO MUCH Fat in your diet* and you may suffer from leaky gut syndrome, obesity (fat has more than twice the number of calories as protein and carbs), and obesity related diseases. You can suffer from clogged arteries depending on the type of fats you are eating. More is not always better!

You should AVOID:

- SATURATED FATS: butter, shortenings, and lard
- TRANS FATS: vegetable shortenings, margarine, crackers, cookies, snack foods, and other foods made with or fried in Partially Hydrogenated Oils (PHOs).

*NOT ENOUGH Fat in your diet* and you will NOT absorb four *ESSENTIAL* vitamins (A, D, E, K), and consequently other minerals and vitamins that rely on the absorption of those four. For example, calcium is not absorbed in a usable form by the body without vitamin D. If you are not getting vitamin D and/or calcium, then your bones will suffer, leading to osteopenia and osteoporosis. You will also experience slow digestion, constipation, and fatigue.

**CARBOHYDRATES:** CARBS are the most important source of energy for the body, especially the brain.

**STOP!**

Back up.

DID YOU SEE THAT?

**CARBS - _THE "BAD GUY"_ – ARE THE MOST IMPORTANT SOURCE OF ENERGY FOR THE BODY! _ESPECIALLY_ THE BRAIN.**

Carbs are the only macro-nutrient that contain fiber and the majority of concentrated vitamins. Your digestive system changes carbohydrates into glucose (blood sugar), which is then used as energy for your cells, tissues, organs, and brain functions.

Carbs are found in vegetables, fruit, grains, nuts, sugar, dairy, breads, pasta, rice, and snack foods.

_TOO MANY Carbs in the diet (in the form of starches and sugar like: desserts, pasta, rice, potatoes, breads, grains, pretzels, crackers, snack foods...) leads to_ insulin resistance, weight gain and obesity, poor digestion, IBS, high cholesterol, Type 2 Diabetes, sluggishness and more.

_NOT ENOUGH Carbs in your diet equals_ low energy, lack of concentration, poor memory, constipation, bad breath, headaches, malabsorption of vitamins and minerals, muscle injury, and weight gain. Yep! You need the right amount of fibrous carbs in your diet to avoid weight gain.

*When you favor one macro-nutrient greatly over the others (and in some cases even eliminating one), you set yourself up for weight gain, nutritional deficiencies, and disease.*

Now, let's get to the JUICY STUFF!

## CALORIES ARE NOT EQUAL

Ok, FOCUS with me for just a minute. We are going to do a little math. I promise it'll be quick and fairly painless. *This is too important to skip because......*

**THIS WILL HELP YOU UNDERSTAND WHY MOST OF YOUR DIET ATTEMPTS ARE EPIC FAILS!**

RECAP - MACRO-NUTRIENTS are:

- Carbohydrates = 4 calories per one gram.
- Proteins = 4 calories per one gram.
- Fats = 9 calories per one gram.
- You must have all three macro-nutrients in your diet to get enough fiber, micro-nutrients, and water.

Let's take three healthy foods in equal amounts and compare:

1) 2 oz. chicken breast (≈1 chicken tender)
   NUTRITIONAL INFO: 58 calories, 2.32g fat, 0g carbs, 8.86g protein

2) 2 oz. Avocado (≈ a little more than 1/4 of a Haas avocado)

NUTRITIONAL INFO: 91 calories, 8.31g fat, 4.84g carbs, 1.13g protein

3) 2 oz. (4 Tbl.) organic natural peanut butter

NUTRITIONAL INFO: 380 calories, 32g fat, 7g carbs, 8g protein

4) Snickers candy bar (regular size ≈ 2 oz.)[24]

NUTRITIONAL INFO: 250 calories, 12g fat, 33g carbs, 4g protein

All of these contain protein, carbohydrates, and fats. But did it surprise you which one had the best calorie count and macro-nutrient ratios?

While the Snickers bar obviously has the least amount of *nutrition,* you can see how **overeating "healthy" foods can lead to WEIGHT GAIN** when compared to the peanut butter and avocado. I know I can eat A LOT more avocado than 2 oz. in a sitting, but I won't eat more than one Snickers bar – not that I'm advocating eating candy over avocados!

> **NOTE:** *We didn't even address alcohol, but remember that alcohol is 2-3 times the number of calories per gram as protein and carbohydrates!*

The point is: **BE AWARE OF PORTIONS, EVEN WHEN EATING NUTRITIOUS FOODS.**

*You can get fat eating healthy food!*

---

24 "Whoever determined that a 1-inch candy bar should be considered 'fun sized' should really evaluate their standards for entertainment." - Someecards

*The key to a successful weight loss plan and a healthy nutritional profile is to know how to choose, prepare and combine the foods that give you the MOST NUTRITION for the FEWEST CALORIES!*

## HOW TO PORTION CONTROL FOR <u>YOUR</u> BODY

*Eat With Your Hands.*

Popular belief is that if you are eating whole foods and plenty of fruits and vegetables, you can eat as much as you want without gaining weight. Don't fall into that trap! I just showed you how this can happen with the previous illustration.

The idea behind that statement is that one cannot possibly eat enough fruits and vegetables to gain weight because they are so low in calories. (16 oz. of raw spinach is only 100 calories.) However, other higher calorie foods also make the "healthy whole foods" list, like avocado (one small avocado is 260 calories), nuts, seeds, nut butter, fatty fish, whole grains, dried fruits, honey and agave, olives, coconut and olive oils, etc. Even some fruits and veggies are high in calories like yucca root, corn, potatoes, dates, bananas, and pineapple. While very nutritious, these higher calorie foods make up the bulk of most peoples' diets. Therefore, PORTION CONTROL IS CRITICAL (even with fibrous green veggies) for weight control and overall health. Too much fiber is no fun either.

Weight control is classified by *weight loss* as well as *weight maintenance*. **How much should you eat?** It is different for everyone depending on their size, activity level, age, gender, and genetic makeup. However, for the average, moderately exercising individual there is an easy way to estimate how much protein, carbohydrates, and fat YOU specifically should eat at each meal.

*Use YOUR hand as your guide.*

The amounts of foods will be proportionate to *your size and frame* if you measure foods using to YOUR OWN HAND instead of generalized items like a baseball or deck of cards. If you are very active you may need to slightly increase your portions.

> **NOTE:** Continue to weigh yourself to make sure you are not over-estimating your calorie needs. If you are gaining weight despite high levels of exercise, then you are eating too much.

Here's how it works:

**PROTEIN:** (chicken, fish, steak, eggs...)
Use the palm of your hand to determine the size and thickness of protein.

**FRUIT:** (limit high calorie fruits for weight loss: bananas, pineapple, mango, dates...)
You should be able to hold the piece of fruit in your hand with a loosely closed fist.

**STARCH and GRAINS:** (includes potatoes, rice, oats, squashes, corn, breads, beans...)
Use the size of your palm again. If you are trying to lose weight or stabilize blood sugar, pick BREAKFAST and/or SUPPER to incorporate these foods. Aim for more fibrous veggies to fill your plate at lunch (this will help with mid-afternoon fatigue).

**VEGGIES:** Use your entire open hand to size up your vegetables. If you are eating fresh leafy greens (salad greens), you can use both hands, but remember to keep the portions in check. Two giant handfuls of raw greens can be problematic for some to digest.

**FATS:** (nuts, nut butters, seeds, olives, avocado, oils, butter, coconut...)
1-2 thumb-sized portions.

## DON'T SKIMP ON CARBS!

I touched on the importance of incorporating carbohydrates along with protein and fat in your diet for life-long health and weight loss. I'd like to get a little more specific about the important role of fiber in a balanced diet. Let's begin with the "bad guy," carbohydrates – my favorite and probably yours too, even if you have shunned them from your shopping cart recently.

Carbohydrates serve as an important role in our body's energy, digestion, and brain function. They are a vital nutrient that we must incorporate into our nutrition plan *daily* for not only our bodies to function properly, but our minds as well. All the body's systems (muscles, organs) run on proteins, fats, and carbohydrates, but the **brain runs on ONE source of fuel: GLUCOSE** (from carbohydrates).

*If you are eliminating or eating too few carbohydrates*, you will experience "BRAIN FOG" which can lead to:

- forgetfulness
- lack of concentration

- mistakes at work or school

- irritability

- and the worst......being HANGRY!

We've all experienced the carb-deprived irritability of ourselves and others. I like to say to the road-ragers out there driving, "Hey! Go eat some carbs!"

Now, before you start the "Fight Road Rage. Eat a Donut" campaign because *"Kim said to eat carbs!! Woo-Hoo!";* let me be specific about *which* carbohydrates I'm encouraging you to eat.

As previously stated, everyone's need for carbohydrates differ depending on their activity, genetics, lifestyle, and personal health. Therefore, you must FIRST figure out how many carbohydrates YOU need in your daily diet by establishing your goals, using your hand for portions, and weighing yourself to see if the scale is going in the direction you desire. Then the fun part begins - EATING.

**Carbohydrates not only give you energy and better focus, but they are also the *only* macro-nutrient that contain FIBER!** Because fiber is not found in protein or fat, you must make sure to incorporate plenty of carbohydrates into your daily nutrition plan.

Carbohydrates should contain as much fiber as possible, but don't overdo it! Too much fiber can cause severe bloating, gas, and digestion issues.

The FDA recommends:

- Men: age 50 or younger should get 38 grams of fiber daily
- Women: age 50 or younger should get 25 grams of fiber daily
- Men: age 51 or older should get 30 grams of fiber daily
- Women: age 51 or older should get 21 grams of fiber daily

DIETARY FIBER — found mainly in fruits, vegetables, whole grains and legumes — is probably best known for its ability to prevent or relieve constipation; a topic we will discuss further later. It's a "bulky" topic.

Foods containing FIBER also provide other health benefits:

- Aid in weight loss
- Help maintain a healthy weight
- Lower the risk of developing diabetes
- Lower the risk of developing heart disease
- Lower cholesterol
- Help maintain healthy blood sugar levels, and more

Dietary fiber, also known as roughage or bulk, includes all parts of plant foods that your body can't digest or absorb. Unlike other food components, such as fats, proteins or refined (white) carbohydrates, which your body breaks down and absorbs, fiber isn't digested by your body. Instead, it passes relatively intact through your stomach, small intestine, colon, and out of your body.

**FIBER** is commonly classified as **SOLUBLE** (it dissolves in water) or **INSOLUBLE** (doesn't dissolve):

- SOLUBLE FIBER: This type of fiber dissolves in water to form a gel-like material. It can help lower blood cholesterol and glucose levels. Some sources of soluble fiber are oats, peas, beans, apples, pears, citrus fruits, carrots, barley and psyllium.

- INSOLUBLE FIBER: This type of fiber promotes the movement of food through your digestive system and increases stool bulk. So, it can be of benefit to those who struggle with constipation. Good sources of insoluble fiber include whole-wheat flour, wheat bran, nuts, beans, and vegetables such as cauliflower, dark leafy greens, green beans and potatoes.

Fiber helps stabilize blood sugar, keeps you full, and aids in digestion. Selecting tasty foods that provide fiber isn't difficult. Most plant-based foods, such as oatmeal and beans, contain BOTH SOLUBLE and INSOLUBLE FIBER. However, the amount of each type varies in different plant foods. Nuts, nut butters, whole grains, and seeds are all good sources of fiber, *BUT* they are also HIGH in calories. So, opt for lower-calorie fibrous veggies and fruits like spinach, apples, green beans, peppers, jicama, berries, etc. to fill you up without filling you out.

Some say money makes the world go 'round. Others say it's love. I believe love makes the world go 'round, but fiber definitely helps! **To receive the greatest health benefit**, eat a wide variety of high-fiber foods, and by all means, enjoy carbs! They're good for your health......and road rage.

## MAKING IT WORK FOR YOU AND YOUR FAMILY

**NOW YOU KNOW WHAT TO EAT, HOW TO EAT, AND HOW MUCH TO EAT.** Your question becomes "How do I make this work for me and my family? How do I incorporate all these foods into a diet plan that works?"

The answer is very simple and yet complex.

*IF GOD MADE IT, EAT IT. IF MAN MADE IT, TOSS IT.*

That seems simple enough until you get home from the grocery store with sacks full of fresh fruits and veggies, meat, chicken, fish, gluten free bread (we'll talk about this later!!), rice, eggs, oats, and a *deer caught in headlights* look on your face.

Here comes the more complicated part. You've just realized that you have all the ingredients to cook an "I HAVE NO CLUE" meal. It's overwhelming to figure out what to do with all this beautiful, fresh God-made food. So, you shove it in the refrigerator to "deal" with later. Maybe you'll try one of those recipes you found on Pinterest. Next Thursday.

Seven days, two soccer games, three school projects, and one stomach bug later, you still haven't "dealt" with all that food you bought. What do you do? You hit the drive-thru because it's faster, easier, and one less thing you have to think about. Until your blood work comes back revealing high blood pressure, high cholesterol, high triglycerides (which you've never heard of before), and a request from your doctor to "come in immediately to discuss the prescriptions" you will now be required to take three times a day. Yep, your list just got longer and more expensive.

*"Tell me what to do, already!" you say?*

If you are used to eating out most of the time or purchasing pre-packaged meals like Lean Cuisine from the grocery store, then

## *DO NOT BUY FRESH PRODUCE, MEATS AND FISH AT THE STORE.*

Let me clarify....

If you cook occasionally and have cooking skills, then *please* buy fresh produce, meats, fish, etc.

But **if you do NOT know how to cook**, you need to start with more simple meal-prep ideas and take cooking classes to help you learn *how* to cook – and cook healthy! You need more education to help you be successful at incorporating fewer processed, more nutritious food into your diet. Don't fret. Cooking classes can be fun entertainment for the whole family. You can even find online classes if you feel time is a factor.

**IT'S A JUGGLING ACT:**

*Start with learning how to SHOP.*

Finding the time to eat healthy, much less cook, can be a challenge for many families these days, when we are already juggling family, work, school, church, and exercise. How can we possibly find time for one more thing? Our hectic, busy lives aren't always conducive to eating balanced nutritious meals. Add the intimidation of a raw chicken staring back at you, and you have a recipe for fast food. Pardon the pun.

Although fast food restaurants are promoting changes in their menus and claiming to have your health in their best interests, obesity continues to rise throughout the American population. You do not have to give up the battle of the bulge or compromise your family's health. **Making nutritious meals** can be **EASY**, and believe it or not, **FASTER** than the drive-thru **if you know how to SHOP!**

I'll be the first to admit that grocery stores can be intimidating. Although I *love* shopping for food like some girls love shopping for shoes, every time I go to a new store, it takes some work and time figuring out the "lay of the land." *If you will shop when you have time instead of between picking up kids or after work when you're starving and don't have a clue what to fix for supper, you will eliminate most of your confusion and frustration.* Set aside a specific day of the week when you can spend some time learning the layout of your grocery store and take your time.

People ask me all the time about *how to read food labels.* This is important, and a great tool, but **if you are NEW to the "healthy" eating lifestyle, then KEEP IT SIMPLE**. If you can't tell what it is, then don't buy it. If there is a long list of unpronounceable words in the ingredients list, then leave it on the shelf. There are no labels on fruit, veggies, cuts of meat, eggs, etc. You catch my drift here. You can find most of these foods *prepackaged* and *precooked* (like salads, guacamole, mixed fruit bowls, hummus, rotisserie chicken...) in your grocery store. Grocery stores have done a lot of the work for you.

You can find these whole, nutritious, REAL foods in the FROZEN FOODS SECTION of the store as well (like frozen rice, sprouted grain breads, quinoa, fruit etc.) ready for you to heat in the microwave. Frozen foods are convenient, readily available, easy to store and prepare, and will not perish as quickly as fresh options. They also don't have the preservatives and chemicals you find in the highly processed, packaged foods.

If trying to figure out what to buy is still causing you heart palpitations, look for classes to help you. (I offer a *Grocery Shopping Tour* for clients where we meet at the grocery store and shop together, as well as online *Healthy Cooking Classes*.)

Learn to love shopping for groceries! If you look around in the produce section, it's really a beautiful array of colors!

## WHAT'S THE BIG DEAL?

# Why is Cooking and Eating at home important?

We've all heard the saying "abs are made in the kitchen." While that is true, I would add that health and longevity also start in the kitchen. Eating is something we must do every day, and one of the few things adults *can control*. We like to think we can't control our cravings and what we eat. However, unless Ronald McDonald himself is holding you hostage and force-feeding you Happy Meals, *you control* what you put in your mouth. Sometimes a lack of knowledge about nutrition or a lack of skills in the kitchen can hinder one's healthy eating plan, but educating yourself in nutrition and learning how to cook is a skill that you will master in time and *take with you for the rest of your life.*

> **SIDE BAR:** If you really want to get a young adult (newlywed, high school or college graduate) a gift they will appreciate, will continuously benefit them, and use for the rest of their lives; sign them up for cooking classes!

Why learn to cook for yourself?

Here are a few reasons cooking at home is beneficial:

➢ *You control the quality of the ingredients.* Not all food products are created equal. If you are purchasing the foods to cook, you can choose products that do not have chemicals, pesticides, highly processed trans fats, sugar, artificial sweeteners, colors, fillers, and other harmful additives.

➢ *You control the calories and portions.* We are all tempted to overeat because of the enormous portions offered at restaurants, but you have the option of only preparing what you will eat in one sitting.

➢ *You can extend family time and make memories.* By cooking at home, you get to include ALL family members. So, you can not only eat together but also cook together. Many life lessons are taught and learned in the kitchen. Some of the most precious memories I have of my Granny is cooking with her. I still use her old pots while teaching my cooking classes today.

➢ *You can be creative!* Cooking is an art form just like painting, sculpting and composing. If you need a creative outlet, use food! Fresh produce is a vibrant palate you can color your plate with while improving your health.

➢ *Kids will try new foods.* Kids are more likely to eat something they cooked or prepared themselves even if they are finicky eaters.

> *Cooking teaches kids and adults how to make healthier choices.* It's a perfect venue to help visualize and understand where vitamins come from and their importance to the health of our bodies. Different colors equal different vitamins and minerals.

> *Cooking is an applicable teaching tool for kids.*

>> ○ They will learn, apply, and perfect math skills like counting, measuring, fractions, etc. without boring worksheets. They will see how math is something they will use in the "real world." (That was our argument as kids for not liking a subject. I'm guessing it still is.)

>> ○ Kiddos learn to read and apply what they read, by following instructions. All of which are imperative in being successful in school and life. Recipes are usually very specific, and if you don't follow the directions precisely, you can end up with a very different result. Cooking is a great hands-on application in understanding and applying what they've read.

>> ○ It teaches focus and discipline. We cannot get distracted or we run the risk of burning our meal.

**"What's for supper?"** may be the number one question asked daily. For some it's an easy answer; "Whatever fast food place is on the way home." But for those who are trying to better their health by eating and cooking meals at home, it can stir up stress and pressure if they don't know *how* or *what* to cook.

Avoid stress by....

### SETTING YOURSELF UP FOR SUCCESS!

Even if you have the skills and enjoy cooking, trying to cook every week night is not realistic for many of you. I love cooking and teach public cooking classes, but even I don't cook every night. I allow some wiggle room, especially during my busy seasons.

*If you want to start cooking at home, try these strategies so you won't feel overwhelmed and give up before you ever get started.*

1) Plan on cooking one to five nights a week. Whatever your schedule and ability allow. Be conservative at first and work your way up to cooking 5 days a week.

2) Plan your menu ahead of time. Pick a day of the week when you will:

   a. plan your menu

   b. write your grocery list

   c. go to the grocery store

3) K.I.S.S. - **K**eep **I**t **S**imple & **S**atisfying. You don't have to cook five course gourmet meals! Choose simple recipes that you and your family will enjoy that don't take a lot of time to prepare. Crock pots are a cook's best friend! Just sayin'.

4) Plan for leftovers. I always teach in my cooking classes that if I'm already doing the work, I might as well double (or triple) the recipe. You can either eat the same meal twice for supper or have it for lunch the following day. Or, my favorite, freeze it for later in the month. If you do this for one meal a week, at the end of each month you will have a week's worth of meals in the freezer, and you won't have to cook at all that week!

However, if you are **NOT** interested in cooking OR want to start eating better **TODAY,** there are some things you can incorporate RIGHT NOW that will significantly improve your current diet while you work your way through the nutritional learning curve.

## WEIGHTLOSS and NUTRITION TIPS YOU CAN INCORPORATE TODAY!

This is a quick look at changes that are easy to make RIGHT NOW with little effort or forethought.

1) **Drink more H20.** Aim to drink at least half of your body weight in ounces of water daily. For example, a 120-lb. person should aim for at least 60 oz. of water daily. If drinking water throughout the day is challenging for you, try writing times on your water bottles with a marker. That way you will see at 9 am, 12 pm, 3 pm, 6 pm you should be drinking that bottle. This makes it easier to keep track, ensures you drink water throughout the day, and holds you accountable.

2) **Eat and be satisfied with smaller portions.** Our portions are out-of-control! Portion size matters most when it comes to proper digestion, weight management, weight loss, or weight gain. For some, several small meals a day works best for proper digestion - their stomachs are not capable of easily digesting large amounts of food at one time. Others do best eating three larger meals a day as frequent snacking is not possible with their schedules. Neither strategy is better than the other; the key is eating the proper portions for YOUR body size and lifestyle.

3) **Food Prep Tips That Make Life Easier....**

Whichever meal timing strategy you use, food prep is key to ensure you are getting proper portions and healthy nutrition throughout the day. I know it can be overwhelming if you have a demanding job, aren't home very often, or don't have a lot of time to cook. Luckily, there are several ways to make eating healthy easier by prepping food ahead of time. Here are a few of my go-to food prep tips:

- **Pre-bake foods** like sweet potatoes, chicken, fish, and roasted veggies in large batches beforehand so that you have three to five days' worth of easy, healthy options to choose from.

- **Make large portions** of healthy grains like quinoa and rice so that you have easy, healthy carbs on hand.

- **Pre-cut veggies** like bell peppers, carrots, broccoli, and cauliflower so that they're easy to grab for snacking, salads, or quick stir fries. OR even better still, buy them pre-cut at the grocery store!

- **Veggie soup** is an easy way to have a snack or quick meal packed full of nutrition. Toss leftovers into a crock pot with some broth and cook it on low all day. To make it more of a substantial meal, add leftover chicken, rice, and potatoes. This can be a life saver when you get home late and need a light meal before bed.

- **Plastic storage containers** and baggies allow you to portion out and pack food ahead for quick lunches and snacks.

4) **Learn to love leftovers!** Seriously, start getting in the habit of making twice as much as usual for dinner; make

enough oatmeal for the next few mornings; make extra of a recipe and freeze the rest for later. That way, when you have zero time to cook, you'll always have something quick and healthy to grab. It makes life so much easier.

- ○ If you eat at a restaurant, bring some food home for lunch the next day. Hopefully, you are ordering nutritious meals!!

- ○ Learn to let the grocery store help you. More and more grab-and-go healthy options are available to you at the grocery stores.

5) **Schedule your meals.** For example: breakfast at 8:00 am, lunch at noon, snack at 4:00 pm, dinner at 7:00 pm. Make your schedule work for your lifestyle. It's important to train your body to eat and sleep on a regular schedule especially if you are having blood sugar, thyroid or hormone issues.

- ○ Label your containers and baggies with the meal and time to eat it so that when you hit the fridge or pack your meals for the day you can spot it quickly. Setting an alarm on your phone to buzz you when it's time to eat is also helpful for many who have busy schedules or forget to eat. It is simple, yet effective!

- ○ Going too long (more than 5 hours) without eating will lead to blood sugar crashes, fatigue, poor concentration, irritability, and overeating (usually junk food) late in the day and night.

- ○ Grazing all day will leave you feeling unsatisfied, lead to overeating, and ultimately weight gain.

6) **Color your plate.** It is no secret that eating a variety of colorful food provides vitamins, minerals, and antioxidants to nourish your body that can't be replicated in a supplement or multivitamin. Hmmm, this keeps coming up. Must be important!

   **Each color contains its own nutrients:**

   - Red: lycopene and anthocyanins
   - Orange: vitamin C, carotenoids, and bioflavonoids
   - Yellow: nutrients that promote good digestion and optimal brain function
   - Green: lutein and indoles
   - Blue/Purple: antioxidants and anti-aging properties
   - White: nutrients that increase immunity

7) **Exercise.** Whether you're lifting weights at a gym, running, or doing body weight exercises at home, exercise will help you build lean muscle and increase bone density. Not only will toned muscle help you look better, but it will make your body a fat burning machine!

8) **Walk daily after dinner.** Making a habit of taking a stroll after dinner helps you unwind, aid digestion, sleep better, get your sunshine (if it's not after dark), and spend a little more family time together.

9) **Clean up.** Rid your home of all the foods that are distracting you from reaching your goals. Notice I did not write "bad" foods. If you cannot control yourself with almond butter, which is a healthy food, then DON'T have it around! You can donate all unopened food items to the

food bank or other charitable organization or give it to a neighbor.

10) **Pick a day of the week** to go to the grocery store and prep meals for the week. Failure to plan is a plan to fail.[25] The worst thing you can do is be starving and not have healthy food available.

11) **Write it down.** Get a food journal or phone app. *This is a crucial step in your lifelong weight loss goals.* Be diligent in journaling your food, sleep, supplements, medications, exercise, etc. It may be your saving grace at some point in your life. It has been mine.

12) **Make your mealtimes about enjoying the meal** you (or a loved one) has prepared. Do not watch TV, return emails, pay bills, check social media, or return phone calls during meals. Meal time is for eating and enjoying friends and family.

13) **INTERMITTENT FASTING** is great for weight loss as well as weight management for several reasons.

    a. It allows your digestive system to fully digest your food which gives it a break.

    b. Every time you eat, your body releases insulin to aid in digestion. Fasting lowers insulin and raises levels of Human Growth Hormone (HGH) which in turn makes fat – specifically belly fat – more accessible for energy use. In other words, you become a fat burning machine by boosting your metabolic rate up to 14%! (HGH is responsible for muscle and bone growth,

---

25  "By failing to prepare, you are preparing to fail." – Benjamin Franklin

sugar and fat metabolism, regulating body composition, body fluids, and heart function in adults. It spurs growth in children and teens.)

c. When you fast, your body's cells initiate important cellular repair and change the expression of genes, which are both related to longevity and protection against disease.

**NOTE:** Not everyone should practice INTERMITTENT FASTING. You should NOT do Intermittent Fasting if:

- ◦ You are underweight
- ◦ You have or have had an eating disorder
- ◦ You are trying to get pregnant or are breastfeeding
- ◦ You have problems with fertility and/or are trying to conceive
- ◦ You are hypoglycemic

**HOW TO PRACTICE INTERMITTENT FASTING:** I have practiced Intermittent Fasting for many years with great success. Here's how to begin:

- ◦ Eat supper at least three hours before bedtime – which you should do anyway! You will technically be doing the majority of your fast while you are asleep! Yea!

- ◦ Only fast for 10-14 hours. Any longer than 16 hours will lead to a binge later, and you won't reap any extra benefits by doing a longer fast. (I rarely fast more than 14 hours.) So, if you eat your last meal at 8:00pm, you will not eat again until 10:00am. That doesn't sound too terrible, right?

- Continue to drink water when you are thirsty. Always drink a glass of water upon waking no matter what.

- Start slowly at first. It took me a couple of years to work up to 14 hours comfortably. Typically, I fast for 12-14 hours, two to three days a week and 15-16 hours once a month.

- Only practice INTERMITTENT FASTING three to four days per week. You will have better luck sticking with it. More importantly, it will work better for digestive health, metabolism boost, and hormone regulation.

## HOW TO COLOR YOUR PLATE

Most would agree that eating plenty of vegetables and some fruit daily is something we all need to address. But why are these foods so important?

While the focus is usually on lean protein and healthy fats, fruits and veggies are where most of the necessary fiber, vitamins and minerals (*micro-nutrients*) are located that keep your body healthy and functioning properly.

**Why not just take a multi-vitamin and skip eating veggies and fruits, you ask?** Whole foods contain the proper ratio of *micro-nutrients* (vitamins and minerals) in a readily absorbable form. The fiber content of the food acts as the "time-release" ingredient that allows your body the optimal time needed to absorb everything efficiently. Recent research shows that multi-vitamins do not contain the right combinations or usable forms of *micro-nutrients* resulting in your body passing them through your system without getting any benefit.

*In other words, you are literally flushing*
*your money down the toilet.*

It is possible to get all the necessary vitamins and minerals through eating real food, but you must eat a wide variety of fruits and veggies to ensure you're getting everything you need daily.

*How do you know if you are getting enough?*

**COLOR YOUR PLATE!**

A tool I use with clients to determine if they are getting enough vitamins and minerals in their daily diet is a **PHOTO FOOD DIARY**. I encourage you to try this method, too.

Here's how:

1) For one day, take a picture with your phone of EVERY meal/snack you eat and drink – everything that goes into your mouth.

2) At the end of the day, take note of how many colors were on your plate.

   a. Was your food mainly brown or white (as in meat, potatoes, grains)?

   b. Or did you have largely *"green"* as your veggie color?

While *"green"* is good, you need ALL colors of the rainbow to make sure you get all the necessary vitamins and minerals your body needs daily - and I'm not talking about Skittles! The more vibrant the color, the more micro-nutrients the food contains.

**An easy way to make sure you're getting plenty of COLOR on your plate every day** is through SOUPS and *BLENDED*

SMOOTHIES *(NOT JUICED SMOOTHIES – more on juicing later)*.

There are times I cannot always eat enough (or any) fruits and veggies. Maybe I'm traveling, don't have time to get to the store and/or cook, or I'm just not very hungry that day.

When those situations arise I always have the following available:

- homemade veggie soup* OR organic canned veggie soup
- green smoothies*
- snack packs: carrots, sugar snap peas, cherry tomatoes, jicama, apple slices

*You can find these recipes and more at*
www.getfitwithkimtoday.com

By focusing on coloring your plate, you will not only get all the *micro-nutrients* you need but also plenty of fiber, which will help you in your weight loss (and poopy) efforts.

## I'M HUNGRY ALL THE TIME!!

There are many reasons you feel hungry all the time. It is possible to turn "off" those hunger signals if you can first figure out what is causing your extreme hunger.

Here are a few basic reasons why you're plagued with constant, ravenous hunger and strategies to help you turn OFF your hunger response:

➢ **You eat when you are stressed or anxious.** There are other emotional reasons people eat, but stress and anxiety can cause your body to go into the "fight or flight" response, which releases cortisol and the "hungry" hormone, Ghrelin.

**THE FIX:**

- First, address the stress and anxiety in your life. Do what is necessary to reduce and ultimately eliminate (if you can) those factors contributing to your stress and anxiety. Then, find other ways of coping other than eating, like exercise, meditation, quiet time, or journaling.

- Try deep breathing right before you eat a meal.

Here's how:

> » Inhale through your nose for five counts
>
> » Hold the breath for three counts
>
> » Exhale through your mouth *completely* in two counts
>
> » Repeat for 5-10 breaths

The act of breathing and counting will relax you by distraction (the counting) and oxygenating the brain (breathing). This also works well if you frequently experience anxiety attacks.

- Have an "EXERTIZER." Instead of an appetizer before a meal, try doing one to two minutes of intense exercise, like jumping jacks, burpees, high knees, or squat hops. The high intensity will literally kill your appetite, giving you an opportunity to avoid the binge, or wait until it's time to eat a proper meal. Plus, it will boost your metabolism, giving you an extra calorie burn.

➢ *Your exercise routine is inefficient.* If you are *over-exercising*, you will be hungrier. *It does not matter if you are doing cardio or weight training.* Exercise of any kind will break your body (muscles) down, and food helps rebuild them stronger and capable of more work. That's how exercise works. Your body is smart and knows it needs food to rebuild. Therefore, it will signal your hunger *stimulating* hormone (Ghrelin) to kick-start, so you will recognize the need to eat.

For those who do SPORADIC and INCONSISTENT workouts (primarily weight training), you will find that you are NOT reaping the benefits of exercise and only making yourself HUNGRY.

**Only moderately exercising two to three times a week (on your own or with a trainer) will do nothing but make you extremely hungry**. It will NOT benefit strength or weight loss efforts. If you give in to that hunger, you will gain weight despite your exercise program.

**THE FIX:**

- Do not do loooonnngg hours of exercise or "two-a-days" unless you are training for an endurance sport.
- Keep workouts focused, intense, and short. Unless I'm training for triathlon, my workouts are 15-50 minutes, MAX.
- You should do purposeful exercise six days a week.
- BE CONSISTENT: If your workouts are short and structured properly, then you can do them every day.

➢ *You don't exercise at all.* Structured correctly, exercise suppresses the appetite by producing the hunger *killing* hormone (Leptin) and helps METABOLIZE FAT. High Intensity Interval Training (H.I.I.T.) workouts are great for this.

However, you don't have to spend a lot of time exercising to get the appetite suppressing benefits.

**THE FIX:**

- If you do one to two minutes of intense exercise – like jumping jacks, squat hops, climbing stairs, etc. - whenever you *feel* hungry (when you know you shouldn't technically *be* hungry), you will release Leptin, which will suppress your appetite and deactivate your hunger response. *ALSO KNOWN AS THE "EXERTIZER."

- Incorporate these short bursts of activity throughout your day. It's a great way to get your workout in when you're short on time, while also suppressing your appetite. Plus, this will also efficiently rev-up your metabolism for several hours helping you tap into those fat stores.

- Incorporate H.I.I.T. workouts into your exercise routine one to two times a week.

➢ *You regularly eat foods containing too much SUGAR or foods with HIDDEN SUGAR.* The hunger associated with sugar is two-fold.

1) Sugar is devoid of any, and all, nutrition. That's why it's called "empty calories." When you eat a lot of sugar, your blood sugar peaks and crashes causing you to need a pick-me-up, which stimulates your hunger response.

2) Because sugar has no nutrition (vitamins, minerals, fiber) your body recognizes that you have not met those needs and will tell you to keep eating until those needs are met. Hence, making you HUNGRY ALL THE TIME. (This response is even worse for artificial sweeteners.)

## THE FIX:

- First, stop eating sugar laden foods.

- Second, rid your house of the problem: all tempting candy, cakes, cookies, drinks

- If you have *over-indulged in sugar* (for example, eating Halloween candy) *for a short period of time* and now you are suffering from SUGAR INDUCED HUNGER, here's what you do:

  » For however many days you indulged, (ex: three days) do the following for the same amount of time (ex: three days):

    ◊ Do not eat any sugar or foods/condiments containing: sugar, honey, agave, stevia etc.

    ◊ Do not eat any fruit. While fruit is a great nutritious way to curb your sweet tooth normally, eating it when you are suffering from SUGAR INDUCED HUNGER will only keep the insanity going!

    ◊ Do not eat STARCHY carbohydrates. Again, the same is true here as with the fruit. Eliminate oats, breads, corn, tortillas, rice, pasta, and white potatoes. While the whole grain versions of these foods are healthy normally, they will also keep the crazy train on the track.

» Once you've done your "time" (ex: three days), start incorporating healthy fruits, veggies (potatoes and corn), and grains (starchy carbohydrates) back into your diet.

○ If you **regularly indulge in sugar** (daily or most days for a month or more):

» You need to address your total nutrition profile.

» I recommend you go on an *Elimination-Reintroduction Diet, but only if you hire a certified nutritionist to guide you through this type of diet.* This is not something that is easily done on your own. The addiction to sugar and the sugar-induced hunger response is just too strong to go it alone. The knowledge a certified nutritionist brings will support your success. [26]

➢ *Eating a diet high in starchy carbohydrates* (breads, pasta, rice, potatoes, corn, tortillas, crackers, chips, popcorn, pretzels, wraps, corn) *will cause you to suffer similar sugar induced hunger pains as when eating foods high in table sugar.* While many of these carbohydrates (grains, oats, rice, potatoes, corn) have some good nutrition (vitamins, minerals, fiber) they can still *stimulate* and *simulate* the sugar induced hunger response *if eaten in excess or too frequently.*

---

26   "A change in bad habits leads to a change in life." – Jenny Craig

**THE FIX:**

> ◦ Follow the exact same recommendations and guidelines outlined above regarding sugar.

➢ *Your diet is comprised of highly processed foods and artificial sweeteners.*

**THE FIX:**

READ FOOD LABELS. I'm not opposed to all packaged foods. Although, *most* everything that comes in a box, wrapper, or can is highly processed. A good rule of thumb when buying packaged foods is to look at the ingredients label on the back. There should be no more than five ingredients, and they should all be food. When the list gets 20 ingredients long and you can't recognize or pronounce most of them, then that's the second clue it's highly processed and full of junk. (The first clue is that it's in a package!) The fewer chemicals, colors, artificial ingredients and sweeteners you eat, the less you will crave them. Focus on incorporating more real, whole foods and fewer packaged foods into your diet.

➢ *Your taste buds are desensitized* due to consuming too many highly-processed foods, salt, sugar, and artificial sweeteners.

**THE FIX:**

RETRAIN YOUR TASTE BUDS!!!

We are born with predominately *either SALTY or SWEET* taste buds. It's genetic. YOU CAN'T CHANGE IT. You will either be predominately drawn to sweet foods or salty foods, but NOT both.

**SIDE BAR:** This is not to say that after eating Mexican Food at your favorite restaurant you won't crave a sweet dessert. We have all been on the roller coaster ride where you eat pretzels (salt) and then need ice cream (sweet) only to crave chips (salty) and then a candy bar! This is the sign that your body is trying to find homeostasis (balance) because you are over-indulging.

While you cannot change the fact that you are born with one or the other, you can significantly *desensitize* your taste buds, so you don't crave either sweet or salty foods *as strongly. It is possible all your cravings will STOP or be greatly reduced by retraining your taste buds. WOOHOO!!* This was life changing for me, coming from a long line of plate-licking pie lovers!

Little known facts about your taste buds:

- They are *VERY sensitive* to artificial sweeteners. Artificial sweeteners make sugar taste bland to your taste buds.

- *In 10 days,* all withdrawal symptoms (from artificial sweeteners, caffeine, sugar, salt) dissipate.

- *In 14 days,* your taste buds begin to "roll over." Food starts to taste like it's supposed to taste, and artificial sweeteners will taste too sweet. *Take my word for it. If you go back to artificial sweeteners at this point, you will have to start the process over. Ugh!

- *In 30 days,* your old taste buds slough off.

- *In 45 days,* you have grown all *NEW* taste buds. Food will naturally taste very sweet and salty without needing to add condiments, sugar, salt, or artificial sweeteners (which will taste bitter with a chemical aftertaste).

Is that not the coolest thing you have ever read?! Let me share it again.

**IN ONLY 45 DAYS**
**YOU CAN RETRAIN YOUR TASTE BUDS**[27]
**AND STOP YOUR CRAVINGS**

# MIC DROP!

➢ *You are eating too frequently. Eating Stimulates Hunger.*

**THE FIX:**

- **Ditch the idea that** you must eat five to eight times a day to "keep your metabolism burning." Or if you don't eat every two to three hours your metabolism will stop, and you will start burning muscle.

## THAT IS JUST NOT TRUE!!
*EATING STIMULATES HUNGER!*

- Quit snacking. It leads to you not eating enough of all the food groups and macro-nutrients (protein, fats, and carbohydrates) at mealtime.

- Eat properly portioned MEALS four to five hours apart. Be sure each meal is complete; containing protein, fat, and carbohydrates according to your personal needs (refer to the portion control section). Research shows that obese people lose significantly more weight when they eat three meals (and possibly

---

27  "When you want something you've never had, you have to do something you've never done." - Unknown

one snack mid-afternoon) as opposed to eating several "mini" meals a day.

- ○ Practice intermittent fasting two to four days a week.

➤ ***Your hormones are out-of-whack.*** There are many hormones that affect hunger and weight. Below are some of the most common.

    a.  Leptin

    b.  Ghrelin

    c.  Cortisol

    d.  Thyroid

    e.  Sex hormones (estrogen, testosterone, progesterone)

**THE FIX:**

Without blood work testing your hormones, you cannot know for certain if those are imbalanced and the root cause of your hunger. Recommendations for what to ask your doctor to check are found in the FAITH section.

*START WITH THE SIMPLEST EXPLANATION, FIRST.*
*More often than not, it*
*REQUIRES THE SIMPLEST SOLUTION TO FIX THE ISSUE!*

Start with your workout routine, lack of exercise, nutrition/diet, and retraining your taste buds *before* taking supplements or rushing to the doctor for Thyroid medicine.

# NATURAL APPETITE SUPPRESSANTS AND METABOLISM BOOSTERS:

1) CINNAMON: suppresses your appetite and:

   a. stabilizes blood sugar

   b. is an anti-inflammatory

   c. boosts metabolism

   d. reduces the need for sugar or sweetness in foods because it activates the same senses on the "sweet" taste buds.

2) HOT PEPPERS and SPICES: The spice and health benefits come from a naturally occurring chemical in peppers called capsaicin. Eating these will:

   a. raise metabolism (the rate at which your body burns calories) up to 23% for 3 hours after eating them

   b. lower cholesterol

   c. relieve pain and inflammation

   d. be useful in treating and preventing some cancers

   e. aid digestion

   f. elevate mood

   g. prevent and clear sinus congestion, ease sinus pain and headaches, and provide pain relief from migraines and cluster headaches

   h. help to reduce the amount of insulin required by diabetics by up to 60%

   i. (one chili pepper) provides more vitamin C than the average orange

3) COFFEE: the unsweetened and dairy-free variety is:

   a.  an appetite suppressant

   b.  full of anti-oxidants

   c.  shown to boost mental and physical performance due to the caffeine

4) GREEN AND HERBAL TEAS

   a.  aid in digestion (primarily peppermint and licorice tea)

   b.  boost metabolism

   c.  are full of anti-oxidants

   d.  appetite suppressant

   e.  regulate blood sugar

   f.  boost immunity

   g.  have anti-inflammatory properties

   h.  reduce water retention

   i.  aid in detoxification

5) NEGATIVE FOODS: These foods take more energy to digest than calories they contain. Incorporating these foods into your diet causes more calories to be burned during digestion than when you eat foods like chicken or potatoes.

   Here are a few:

   a.  Bok choy

   b.  Celery

   c.  Cucumbers

d. Bitter greens: kale, chard, mustard greens, collards, spinach etc.

e. Jicama

f. Grapefruit

g. Lemons and limes

h. Cabbage

i. Broccoli

j. Apples

## MORE ON SUGAR

Fall is the beginning of the holiday season, and for many, a candy "crush." (This is my problem area. I love candy!) 'Tis the season for cooler weather, football, Halloween, Thanksgiving, CANDY, and let's not forget the Pumpkin Spice Latte from Starbucks!

There's much to be thankful for, and even more to enjoy with the coming of Fall, but all too often it also begins our battle with the bulge. Everywhere you look there's candy – even in your own pantry. After all, we don't want the stores to run out by Halloween and be stuck with nothing for the trick-or-treaters. The Pumpkin Spice Latte is seasonal, and we MUST get it while we can!

Yep, I fall for that logic, too. So, what's so bad about enjoying a sweet treat every now and then anyway? Well, it depends on whether it's more "now" and less "then."

Here are a few surprising effects sugar has on your body and health:

These we know:

- Cavities and gum disease
- Weight gain (and not the good kind!)
- Leads to Type 2 Diabetes
- Leads to heart disease
- Can contribute to rapidly growing cancer cells

But here are some you may not be familiar with:

- Too much sugar sends your hunger hormones into a tailspin tricking your brain into thinking you are not full, and your body feels like you have not eaten. The same is true with artificial sweeteners.

- Sugar ages you and makes you look OLDER! How? Oxidative stress turns our tissues "brown" - known as the Maillard reaction. So, in a sense, we "rust" with age. Chronically overindulging in sugar will speed up this process.

- It causes *non-alcoholic FATTY LIVER*. Our body turns excess sugar into fat. If you overindulge on a regular basis, the liver can't keep up and has no choice but to add the fat to itself – i.e. Fatty Liver. This in turn causes the pancreas to make extra insulin to help the liver out. An increase in organ fat does NOT necessarily mean you will see it on the outside of your body, either. *According to a 2012 study in the Journal of Clinical Nutrition, people who ate 1,000 extra calories of sugary foods only saw a 2% increase in body weight, but a 27% increase in liver fat. (I keep wanting to add an exclamation point to the end of that statement!!)*

- The result of the pancreas having to step in? INSULIN RESISTANCE.

I don't want to rain on your parade. By all means, have a candy bar once in a while, but watch how much sugar you are actually consuming.

The Lesson Here: *Be mindful of what you eat.*

So many processed foods (even "healthy" foods) have a lot of *added sugars* in them, and it adds up. Save the sweet treats for special occasions, like a birthday or wedding, and you will avoid the negative health issues and weight gain that comes with sugar.

**Here are a few strategies to help you through the candy season:**

- DO NOT buy the *fun size* candy bars thinking that will help you portion control! It's too easy to lose track of how many of those little fat bombs you eat. Instead, buy the regular size and portion it out. You'll eat less. Trust me.

- If you do decide to go the *fun size* candy bar route, set an empty jar next to the candy jar. Every time you eat one, put the wrapper in the jar instead of throwing it away. You'll at least be able to see how many you have eaten that day.

- Better yet, instead of eating the candy, put $1 in the jar every time you pass it up. Give the money you collect to the kids at Halloween. You'll be the favorite house on the block, and you won't run out of candy, either!

**FOOD FOR THOUGHT:**

*How we start the Holiday Season in regard to our eating*
*will determine*
*how we enter the New Year!*

*"You cannot escape the responsibility of tomorrow*
*by evading today."*

*~ Abraham Lincoln*

## THE DANGERS OF "DIET": ARTIFICIAL SWEETENERS

It's in everything from yogurt to gum to bread and even water. We expect to see the "diet" versions of snack foods like cookies, cakes, candy and soft drinks, but when we begin to see our healthy options turning to "diet," it gives me concern.

I am constantly reading labels and researching new foods in the grocery stores. I've become accustomed to seeing the *sugar-free* (or "diet") versions of many *packaged, processed* foods, but one that really got my attention was the variety of waters. You'll find vitamin water, energy water, re-hydrating water (as if good 'ole plain water wasn't getting the job done there!), oxygenated water, and smart water. What's so smart about it? Now if they called it "remember where you put your keys" water, I might actually consider it. But seriously, we do tend to succumb to marketing and advertising just like teenagers succumb to peer pressure.

We all strive for good health and even great health. We are busy and crunched for time, and we will take any edge we can get when it comes to quick and easy meals on the go. We read the labels trying to select the best snacks. In our minds, we go through the list: "Fat is bad; non-fat. Sodium is bad; low-sodium. Calories; not sure what they are but they should be low. Sugar is the worst of them all; *sugar-FREE!* (Or, sweetened with artificial sweeteners)." You've made your choice and feel good about the sugar-free, fat-free, low calorie snack you've selected.

At least you feel good until about 30 minutes after you've eaten it. Now the "fun" begins: hunger pangs, eyeing the vending machine where your favorite chips or candy bar taunts you, headache, uncomfortable bloating, and the dreaded gas – the kind of gas where you literally see your belly growing before your eyes. You fight the urge to eat again, but hunger always wins. So, you head to the vending machine or raid your co-workers secret stash while they're away from their desk. While the guilt sets in about eating again so soon, you opt for the "DIET" (i.e. SUGAR-FREE) snack in efforts to offset the calories, and the vicious cycle begins again.

While there are significant health issues related to ingesting large amounts of refined sugar and high fructose corn syrup, **the artificial sweeteners** saturating the sugar-free and diet foods and drinks **are the culprit for most of your "uncomfortable issues"** (let's call them). *Artificial sweeteners are hindering your weight loss efforts, wreaking havoc on your digestion and contributing to diabetes, heart disease and obesity as well.*

*Frustrated* and *confused* are verbs people commonly use when they come to me with questions about sugar, artificial sweeteners ("fake sugars"), and healthy options for their sweet tooth. Let's address artificial sweeteners.

123

A few of the most popular artificial sweeteners available are:

- **Sucralose** (Splenda): 600 times sweeter than sugar

- **Aspartame** (Nutra Sweet, Equal): 160–220 times sweeter than sugar

- **Saccharine** (Sweet N' Low, Sugar Twin): 200–700 times sweeter than sugar

- **Acesulfame Potassium** (Sunett, Sweet One): 200 times sweeter than sugar

These artificial sweeteners are in almost every "diet" drink, "lite" yogurts, puddings, ice creams, "low-carb" foods, and "reduced-sugar" products including gum. Check out the ingredients list on your favorite SPORTS DRINKS and PROTEIN POWDERS, and you're sure to find them listed there, too.

Because artificial sweeteners are so much sweeter than sugar you are desensitizing your taste buds causing sugar (and fruits) to no longer taste sweet to you. This in turn tricks your brain into thinking all naturally sweet food (like fruit) should come with that astronomical level of "super sweetness," too. Our bodies correlate sweet foods with calories. So, in theory you consume a fraction of a calorie from artificial sweeteners to get the sweetness of many more calories worth of sugar. This sounds like a good weight loss tool, but at what cost?

By desensitizing your taste buds to the true sweetness of natural foods, you trick your brain into thinking it's not only getting 600 times the amount of sweetness, but that calories should also come with that level of sweetness. When you don't get those calories, your appetite and sugar cravings return with a vengeance, and you continue eating/drinking until your body finally gets those expected calories. Since we crave what we eat, what will we crave the next time? When fruits don't taste as sweet due to desensitized taste buds, how will vegetables will taste?

When food isn't palatable, we are NOT going to eat it. Therefore, we are left with the options of more and more sweet "fake" foods like diet drinks, cakes, and candy. Unfortunately, those "fake" foods have *NO NUTRITIVE VALUE* and our *HUNGER will RAGE OUT OF CONTROL* until we feed our bodies the nutrients from real food they crave.

**In fact, those with insulin sensitivity or insulin resistance are at greater risk of increasing those issues by consuming artificial sweeteners instead of sugar.** This vicious cycle can lead to insulin spikes and weight gain, which in turn, increase the risk for developing metabolic syndrome, diabetes, osteoporosis, and cardiovascular problems.

Research has shown that people who drank at least one diet drink a day increased their girth 70% more than those who abstained over a 10-year period, while those who drank two or more saw their belt size grow at a 500% greater rate. A 2011 study showed the same people who drank one diet drink daily increased their risk of heart disease, stroke, heart attack, gout, and blood clots by 61%.

I'm not saying that drinking one diet drink *occasionally* is the culprit for all your health issues or concerns any more than eating that slice of cake on your birthday. Your body is designed to be able to process the occasional unhealthy meal with ease, but you may be unaware of how much "fake sugar" you are consuming *cumulatively* throughout your day if most of your food intake comes in the form of "diet," "sugar-free," or "low-carb" fares.

## Your Defense System:

Your **NUMBER ONE WEAPON** against fighting the bulge, healing your gut (digestive system), and the health risks associated with weight gain is **READING FOOD LABELS.** Arm yourself with knowledge about what's in the foods you eat. When in doubt, choose whole foods, like fresh produce, eggs, fish, meat, nuts, etc. I've never picked a box of food off a tree – if you catch my drift.

Learn to satisfy your daily sugar cravings with fresh fruit, honey, dates, and occasionally, a little stevia. Save your sugar laden treats for special occasions. After all, if you eat it every day, it's no longer a "treat."

> **On a side note:** If you are on the fence about giving up your diet drinks (or whatever "diet" food is a staple for you), I challenge you to give it a try. Eliminate artificial sweeteners from your diet for a couple of weeks and see if your "uncomfortable issues" and cravings subside. I would rather see my clients *occasionally* drink a regular coke than a diet coke because the effects of real sugar are much less severe than the effects of artificial sweeteners. Clear sodas are even better because they don't have the artificial colors. Of course, giving up ALL soft drinks and diet drinks is the best option.

## BELLY BLOAT: Causes and Solutions

Having a flat stomach is on the minds of men and women alike. Sometimes, even the fittest, are attacked by the dreaded belly bloat. Have you noticed that when you wake up in the morning, your tummy is nice and flat, but by the end of the day it looks like you've swallowed a basketball? Not to mention the accompanying pain and discomfort.

Having a bloated stomach is not always a symptom of gas accumulation. While stored fat can be a cause, *most people have other reasons contributing to this problem.*

Your digestive tract may have developed an excess of trapped air due to poor eating habits. Consuming certain foods that are not tolerated causes irritations leading to poor digestion and BLOATING.

## THE MOST COMMON THINGS THAT LEAD TO BELLY BLOAT and HOW TO COMBAT THEM!

### EATING TOO FAST

It's true. Digestion starts in the mouth, and the faster you eat the harder your stomach must work to break down the food. Add eating too much and/or foods that your body doesn't tolerate well, and you've got a recipe for severe bloating, gas, indigestion, and acid reflux (which leads to esophageal erosion and possibly cancer). Plus, if your body is not able to properly digest the foods you eat, then it's impossible for you to get all the nutrients you need from those foods, and your health suffers.

We eat on the run, literally. We don't have time to sit down and enjoy a meal with a friend, much less chew our food 30 times. Our waistlines and health will eventually suffer if we continue on this "gobble it down while we multi-task" eating trend.

Sitting down, thoroughly chewing your food, savoring the meal and the company you share it with, will not only help you avoid the dreaded belly bloat and indigestion, but also slim your waistline. It's proven that those who eat slower consume fewer calories and feel satisfied sooner than those who eat on the run. If you take an OTC or Rx antacid, try chewing your food more thoroughly and see if you can reduce, or possibly eliminate your need for it!

## FOOD INTOLERANCES

**Food intolerances should not be overlooked but investigated. In addition to causing stomach bloating they may cause other health problems.** It is possible for ANY food - including herbs and spices - to be intolerable or an issue for someone. However, most of us do fine with ALL foods, if they're eaten in MODERATION and CHEWED THOROUGHLY.

Some common foods people are allergic to or find intolerable are:

- Dairy
- Wheat gluten
- Nuts
- Eggs
- Shellfish

It's a popular trend right now to eliminate specific foods (wheat for example) even if one does not have a food sensitivity. This is not beneficial long term. While eliminating these more common "intolerable" foods can initially reap some digestive benefits for those who are not sensitive to them, it is a life-saving must for those who *do* have a severe intolerance or allergy to certain foods and additives.

You may need to go on an Elimination-Reintroduction Diet and/or get tested for specific food allergies to see if you have any intolerances to specific foods.

With most of my clients who do NOT have diagnosed food sensitivities or allergies, I find that if they eat these less tolerable foods in MODERATION and CHEW their food WELL, they have NO ISSUES with digestion, gas, bloating, etc. The foods are tolerated just fine.

*If you find that eliminating or reducing specific foods in your diet helps with digestion, bloating, weight loss, etc., take the necessary steps to avoid those foods.*

> **NOTE:** It is possible to develop an intolerance, and even an allergy, to certain foods if you restrict your diet *unnecessarily* for a long period of time. For example, becoming a Vegan for weight loss purposes or following a gluten-free diet when you do not suffer from Celiac Disease.

## PROCESSED FOODS

Processed foods contain high amounts of sodium and other chemicals and additives that can contribute to stomach bloating. Some "healthy" foods (usually labeled as "Lite," "Zero Calorie," "Sugar Free," and "Fat-Free") also contain high levels of harmful ingredients, like artificial sweeteners and oils that cause gas buildup in the stomach.

Avoid processed foods containing high amounts of:

- Sodium
- Artificial sweeteners
- Dyes
- Preservatives
- MSG (monosodium glutamate)
- Soy derivatives
- Hidden sugars and oils

If it comes in a box or a package, and it does not resemble something you would see in nature, it has been processed to some degree – including agave and stevia.

Don't be fooled by the label **"Organic,"** either.
**If it's a box of ORGANIC cookies,
it's still a box of COOKIES!**

Choose natural foods and those you prepare at home as often as possible. Consume more whole foods like fruits, vegetables, lean meats and eggs, and whole grains which are much lower in or completely free of sodium, artificial ingredients, chemicals, fillers, and bi-products.

## EATING RIGHT BEFORE BEDTIME

Supper is the last main meal of the day and should be eaten at least two or three hours before going to bed. It should be something light and easy to digest so you will not be going to bed with a full stomach. Eating right before bed is a mistake that causes weight gain and inflammation in the body by hindering digestion and disrupting sleep: both of which lead to constipation, indigestion, acid reflux, weight gain, and disease.

**If you're frequently hungry right before bed, try these strategies.** But remember, it will take a few days to retrain your hunger signals. Give it at least a couple of weeks to establish these new strategies and make them habits.

- Eat a little more at supper. Try eating an extra serving of colorful veggies. Avoid making your starch (bread, potatoes, rice, pasta) or protein servings bigger, as they take up less room in your stomach than the fibrous veggies. You will feel more satisfied with a fuller tummy by adding more fibrous veggies.

- Take a walk after you eat. Not only will it distract you from the fridge, but will also aid digestion, relax you, and suppress the hunger stimulating hormone, Ghrelin.

- Herbal (specifically peppermint) and sleepy teas are also great to drink before bed because they aid in digestion and help you sleep.

- Try eating an earlier breakfast. You will be less hungry throughout the day and able to eat a lighter supper.

## BE MINDFUL

**Mindless eating** can quickly add inches to your middle, destroying all your good dieting progress. In social situations, where there are more than two of you dining together, the meal typically lasts much longer than usual. In these instances, you may find yourself finishing off the bread basket or chip bowl after eating your meal, while continuing to socialize. Eating in front of the TV or computer with an unlimited portion of food is an equally dangerous form of mindless eating that also leads to bloating, indigestion, and unwanted weight gain.

While a flat stomach is nice, proper digestion and absorption of nutrients is crucial to your health. Maintaining a healthy weight and incorporating the strategies above will not only give you a flatter and more comfortable tummy but also add years to your life!

# DIETS, MYTHS, DETOXES & MORE

# BEFORE YOU GO ON ANOTHER
# DIET, DETOX, OR CLEANSE,
# READ THIS SECTION!

There is no doubt that we live in the age of information – and much of the time, **mis**information. Google any topic, and you can find "evidence" supporting just about any view you want. This is especially true when it comes to health and wellness, diet and nutrition, fitness and exercise. With conflicting arguments for every opinion and a "cure" for any and everything ailing you; too much information and too many viewpoints can be overwhelming, and extremely frustrating for those *WHO JUST NEED HELP.*

Therefore, I'm going to speak a little *TRUTH* about the subject matter that I'm passionate about and educated in: nutrition and fitness (a.k.a. diet and exercise). First of all, I really do not like using the terms "diet and exercise" because that implies there is a one-size-fits-all plan for everyone. *This is just not true.* While yes, the human body technically *should* contain the same working parts inside and out, and *should* work and function in the same ways; everyone is unique in their genetic make-up, environmental influences, personal likes and dislikes, and in their limitations – be it physical, economical, or availability. *These and other factors all contribute to a unique and specific "diet and exercise" profile for every individual.* Therefore, I use the terms *"nutrition" and "fitness,"* respectively.

*One of my hopes for this book is to help you decipher the good information from the bad with truth and tools you can apply to any trendy "diet and exercise" program.*

The truth is, weight loss is a simple process. It requires an energy deficit (fewer calories consumed than burned). There are a few things you need to do to make the process work, but it's not complicated. Since everyone's body and needs are different, it's important to learn which foods *help* and which foods *hinder your personal* weight loss and overall health.

When "QUICK FIX" DIETS restrict food groups, calories, or arrange the macro-nutrients (protein, carbs, and fat) in a way that eliminates or reduces one group drastically, then you are setting yourself up for:

- Disease
- Weight gain!
- Musculoskeletal Injuries
- Digestive issues – IBS, colitis, diverticulitis...
- Developing food intolerances!
- Weakened immune system
- Malnourishment
- AND HUNGER

**STOP!** Did you get all that?

**If you are picking a diet for weight loss**
– which is why most people go on a specific diet –
**you are setting yourself up for eventual WEIGHT GAIN,**
not to mention all the other *crazy* potential side effects
and diseases.

This is the opposite of what we want, but somehow the promise of "quick, effortless weight loss" wins, more often than not.

# BE LEERY OF YOUR FRIEND'S "DIET" OR WEIGHT LOSS "STRATEGY"

I see this happen all the time. Overnight, your coworker or friend shows up looking *A-mazing* and 30 lbs. lighter. (Because weight loss always happens overnight! Ha! It always seems that way for everyone but you though, right?!) Immediately, everyone wants to know the "secret weight loss plan" they stumbled upon. Whether intended or not, they suddenly get thrown into the diet "expert" category.

> **SIDE BAR:** I'm all for sharing information and strategies that help people get healthy!! By all means, if you happen upon a program that gets you long-term results, KEEP DOING IT! My goal is NOT to change anything that's working for you – it's only to help motivate and encourage you to keep going, and possibly help you fill in any gaps to make your program even more successful. This topic is more for those who are still trying to find their way.

Just because your neighbor's teenage pool boy is tan and ripped, doesn't mean we should all go on his diet. First of all, he's 19. They're all ripped! Secondly, he's doing manual labor in the sun. Of course, the pool boy is going to be tan and ripped. It doesn't matter what he eats!

Joking aside, trying every diet that comes across your path is like playing Russian Roulette with your health. You have no idea (and neither does your neighbor) *which foods interact with medications or other conditions*, like thyroid disorders, for example.

*This is detrimental to your health*
*and hinders your progress!*
No one wants that kind of setback.

*The first thing you should always do* is take a step back and evaluate whether the weight loss program is a safe and feasible diet program *for you*. Just because it worked for someone else, DOES NOT guarantee IT'S SUITABLE FOR YOU or that YOU WILL HAVE the same RESULTS. It can actually be VERY DANGEROUS TO GO ON YOUR FRIEND'S "DIET."

Marketing and buzz words can make diets, exercise programs, pills and supplements sound as though they finally found the "magic pill" or "quick fix" of the century. I get sucked in every time, too! I try to always evaluate what's being sold and remind myself that "if it's too good to be true, IT IS!" But I promise, if I find the "magic pill," I'll shoot you a text from the front of the line to get it. Ha!

Be supportive and happy for your friend's success. At the same time, be your own advocate. If you want a truly *safe* and *effective* nutrition program that will help you reach your goals and be something you can maintain for *life*, seek out a professional – a Certified Nutrition Specialist – to help design a program SPECIFIC TO YOUR BODY and your needs.

## THE "ONE SIZE FITS ALL" MENTALITY: COOKIE-CUTTER EXERCISE AND NUTRITION PLANS

When I'm shopping for clothes, and I find something really cute, the first thing I do is look at the label to see what size it is. If the label says, "one size fits all" I just put it back and keep shopping because I know from experience that the label is false. One size *never* fits all – especially me.

Why would an exercise program, diet, aerobics class, personal trainer, or supplement be any different?

*Why do we so often fall victim to COOKIE-CUTTER PLANS?*
**Because every diet or exercise plan has worked for at least one person, and we hope it will work for us, too.**

Unfortunately, it seems we must try several to find the one that *will* work for us. That is why there is a diet and workout plan for anything and everyone.

It's popular for certain exercise cultures to also adopt a specific diet as well. For example, CrossFit uses the Paleo Diet to complement their style of training. While this may work for some people, it will not work for others due to ability, taste preferences, allergies/intolerances to foods, socio-economic limitations, schedule, etc.

*So how do you choose a diet and exercise plan that will work for you without weeding your way through them all?*

When choosing a workout style or trainer, take into consideration whether you have the time and/or resources to do it, if it's something your body can handle, and if the workouts are fun and enjoyable for you. If you don't know how to swim and are fearful of the water, then triathlon may not be your sport. If flipping tractor tires and jumping on boxes sounds like a fun challenge to you, then CrossFit is for you.

Be honest with yourself about your likes/dislikes, commitment level, schedule, and ability about different fitness programs. This will help you *find something that you will stick with and reach your fitness goals.*

**When choosing a nutrition/diet plan, ask yourself these questions to help you find the plan that will work for you LONG TERM:**

- Is it too restrictive? Does it take out entire food groups and/or macronutrients *(protein, fat, and carbs)?* Does it require too few calories? *Eventually, you run out of food and calories to take out, leaving you malnourished, hungry, and yo-yo dieting.*

- Can I afford it? Am I able to eat the way the program recommends on my budget? *Organic is great— unless I can't make my car payment.*

- Is it *real* food based? Or do I have to purchase their food and supplements? *That is a big RED FLAG! I never recommend a program where reliance on their products determines your success. Beware of these diets. I always wonder how they plan on you traveling with an extra suitcase full of their drinks, supplements, and food.*

- Is this plan something I can maintain for life? *If you can't do it for more than 30 days, why would you think you can eat that way for life?*

**Exercise programs** should be fun, but challenging. They

should evolve with your fitness level, challenging your body to become increasingly fit and healthy, *without injury.*

**Diet/nutrition programs** should contain all the macronutrients (protein, fat, and carbs), get your body the proper nutrients (water, fiber, vitamins, minerals, calories), and should fit your personal tastes and special needs. The one-size-fits-all cookie-cutter plans are fine for some, but know that there are OTHER OPTIONS.

## DIET AND WEIGHT LOSS MYTHS

### Drinking water will curb your appetite. <u>TRUE & FALSE</u>

Very few people have a good grasp on the difference between being hungry and being thirsty because the sensations of both are so similar. However, you can retrain your body and your brain to recognize the difference by drinking something instead of eating, and then waiting 15-20 minutes. If you still feel hungry, then eat.

> **TIP:** *Don't stand by the fridge counting down your 15 minutes. Distract yourself!*

While this is all true, *it only works if you are dehydrated.* If you are regularly drinking enough water, then this will not work for you.

Instead, it will cause the opposite effect –
HUNGER and INTENSE CRAVINGS!

**How much is enough?**

Everyone is different, and this is something you need to note in your food journal to figure out what works best for your body. You must take into consideration your activity, the weather, and your sweat rate. A good guideline though is to drink ½ of your bodyweight in ounces throughout the day, and add an additional 8 oz. to that amount for every hour you exercise. (That amount will change if you are exercising in the heat or humidity).

**NOTE:** *As you lose (or gain) weight, your hydration needs change. Therefore, don't forget to recalculate the amounts accordingly.*

## Everyone should eat a GLUTEN FREE diet. <u>FALSE!</u>

Only **1%** of Americans suffer from CELIAC DISEASE, an inherited autoimmune disease that causes damage to the small intestine when gluten (a protein found in wheat) is ingested. Although trendy right now, not everyone HAS TO or NEEDS TO go on a gluten-free diet, even if they are somewhat "sensitive" to gluten.

**Many people who are SENSITIVE to gluten are doing TWO things to CAUSE the sensitivity:**

1) They are eating TOO MANY foods containing gluten (wheat laden carbs – breads, snacks, desserts, pasta, fast foods, processed foods, etc.). If you suffer with *any* food sensitivities, look at what you are eating throughout the entire day. The *PHOTO FOOD DIARY* is perfect for this!

For example, your day may contain some of the following choices:

- Breakfast = cereal, instant oatmeal, toast, or breakfast burrito
- Snack = breakfast bar or meal replacement bar of some sort
- Lunch = sandwich and chips
- Snack = cookies, pretzels, crackers and cheese
- Supper = spaghetti, burrito, casserole, or includes bread/pasta
- Snack = cookie, cereal, chips

This menu overloads the digestive system with gluten. If you ate red meat six times a day, it would cause the same distress. *No matter the food, if you regularly eat too much of anything, a "sensitivity" will develop.*

2) Add the fact that we **barely chew our food before swallowing** to *eating too much* of the "intolerable" food regularly, and we have the perfect storm for food sensitivity. In our hectic, busy lives, we rarely take time to sit down and eat, much less chew our food 30 times before swallowing.

BEFORE eliminating a food from a client's diet, I always have them practice chewing everything thoroughly AND reduce the amount of the "problem" food. Often, this fixes all their issues without having to uproot their lives with a restrictive "YES" and "NO" foods list.

Eat foods containing gluten (breads, pasta, tortillas) in moderation – not even daily – and you will see a reversal or significant reduction in your digestive issues. Do the same with red meat, dairy, and any other food that causes you distress. *Why make yourself miserable and restrict your food if you don't need to?* You may even see significant weight loss, among other things, as a bonus!

**GLUTEN-FREE DOES NOT EQUAL HEALTHY.** Just because a food is labeled "gluten-free" does not mean that it is figure friendly OR good for you. A gluten-free cookie IS STILL A COOKIE!

*The fact is: foods containing gluten - like cookies, cakes, pies, breads, snack foods - should NOT BE A STAPLE in your diet, whether you have Celiac Disease or Gluten Sensitivities or not.*

It's awesome that those who suffer with Celiac have more options available to them. By all means, enjoy the fact that you can have gluten-free cake! (Insert a happy dance here.) Just eat it on your birthday. And invite me over!

## You should buy everything ORGANIC. FALSE

There is a lot of confusion on what to buy organic and if it's even necessary. There's the Dirty Dozen and the Clean Fifteen lists. (You can easily find these online.) There's cage free, free range, non-GMO, grass fed, hormone free, and the list goes on and on.

**First, let's clarify what ORGANIC *is* and *is not*.**

Organic produce is grown without the use of pesticides, synthetic fertilizers, sewage sludge, genetically modified organisms (GMO), or ionizing radiation.

<u>Organic animal products</u> - meat, poultry, eggs, and dairy products – come from animals that do not take antibiotics or growth hormones.

**LABELS:**

<u>100% Organic</u> - Foods bearing this label are made with 100% organic ingredients and may display the USDA Organic seal.

<u>Organic</u> - These products contain at least 95-99% organic ingredients (by weight). The remaining ingredients are not available organically but have been approved by the NOP (National Organic Program).

*Is Organic Produce **more nutritious** than Conventionally Grown Produce?* **NO.**

There is no evidence confirming any nutritional difference between organic foods and those grown conventionally, mainly because it's so difficult to test. The verdict is still out.

*Does Organic Produce **taste better** than Conventionally Grown Produce?*

Taste is subjective, but many people do find that organically grown produce tastes better. It's your call.

**WHAT DO I RECOMMEND?**

*Yes,* there are some foods I *do* buy organic. If you feel better buying and eating all organic, then do it. However, if it's a matter of buying organic food and paying your rent that month, then there's not much of a choice. Let's be realistic. Eating more fruits, veggies, lean meats, eggs, and fish – whether organic or not – is still better than hitting the drive-thru.

**Here are my "RULES" for purchasing ORGANIC. Or NOT:**

- If the food is a STAPLE in my diet - something I (or my hubby) eat or drink every day or most days – then I buy ORGANIC.

> **SIDE BAR:** Sugar is not (and should not be for anyone) a *staple* in my diet. If I'm going to make my Granny's Banana Pudding, I'm not going to use organic sugar because I only make it a couple times a year. I do buy Raw Sugar for my hubby because he puts it in his coffee every morning. I know, I know. But pick your battles. At least raw sugar is not bleached, so I feel better about it.

- If I am going to blend the stems, roots, and/or leaves of a fruit or vegetable into a smoothie, I buy ORGANIC.

- It must be reasonably priced. Sorry, but I'm not spending $50 on an "organic," "cold processed," "yada yada yada" chicken. I find a healthy compromise. When purchasing meat, poultry, and fish I look for "natural"- those raised responsibly without growth hormones or antibiotics, and not processed with fillers or "juice," that's in my price range. (If you buy beef from Texas ranchers, it's free range and grass fed.)

- EGGS: I raise my own chickens and ducks and get fresh eggs daily. I must start with a few facts about chickens.

- CHICKENS ARE OMNIVORES! They eat grain, produce, insects, grubs, worms

- SUNSHINE makes everything and everyone happier. HAPPY CHICKENS ARE HEALTHY CHICKENS.

- The darker yellow-orange the yolk, the healthier the egg. If your egg yolks are pale yellow, buy different eggs.

- Fresh eggs do not have to be refrigerated if you don't wash the shells. They have a protective coating on them that keeps them fresh without refrigeration, unless you wash them!

- Grocery store eggs do need to be refrigerated because they have been processed and washed before they are shipped to the store.

- There is no nutritional difference between white and brown eggs. The type of chicken determines the color of the eggs. I have chickens that lay green and blue eggs!

*Below are what the "labels" on the egg cartons mean. You decide for yourself which to buy.*

- CAGE FREE: the chickens are not kept in a cage, but they are not outside either.

- FREE RANGE: these chickens are not kept in cages and can go outside, but how long they spend outside depends on the farmer.

- ORGANIC: they could be cage free or not. "Organic" means they eat organic feed and do not receive vaccines, hormones or antibiotics.

- VEGETARIAN: the chickens are kept in cages or

indoors. They are fed a vegetarian diet free from meat or fish by-products. They are not allowed outdoors to peck any grubs, worms, or insects. *Remember what I wrote above? Chickens are OMNIVORES.

- ○ PASTEURIZED: these eggs (not the chickens) have been put through a pasteurization process where the egg is heated to 140° without cooking the egg but killing off bacteria. *I recommend pregnant women, the elderly, toddlers under three years old, and those with weakened immune systems (cancer patients) eat *Pasteurized* eggs to reduce the risk of contracting salmonella.

- ○ CONVENTIONAL: these chickens produce your standard grocery store – cheapest – eggs. They are packed into over-filled hen houses and never get outside. They are typically fed a cheap, grain-based diet supplemented with vitamins and minerals, and they are treated with hormones and antibiotics, due to the poor diet and living conditions. NEVER BUY THESE EGGS!!

- ○ OMEGA-3: these are basically like conventional eggs, but have had their feed supplemented with omega-3 containing ingredients – usually flax seed. These chickens rarely get to go outside.

- ○ PASTURED: not to be confused with *pasteurized.* They can roam free eating plants, bugs and insects (their natural food) along with commercial feed.

- • Organic cookies are still cookies. Grass fed beef hamburgers are still hamburgers. Don't fall victim to fancy marketing ploys.

- If it's something that is a once-in-a-while item for us, then I don't bother with the extra expense of buying organic.

- If it's corn or a corn product – chips, tortillas, corn meal, polenta - I *always* buy ORGANIC. Soy and corn are the most Genetically Modified Foods (GMOs) on the planet – Soy being #1. It pays to buy organic with corn.[28]

**SIDE BAR:** I DO NOT RECOMMEND EATING SOY, EVER, FOR ANYONE (especially infants and children under 20 years of age). Even organic soy contains phytoestrogens that mimic estrogen in the body and disrupt the endocrine system. Women who have had or are at risk for developing breast cancer are advised to not eat any soy products for this reason. It can really impact your hormones, especially growing kiddos and those going through adolescence.

Hormones are responsible for regulating many functions in the body - from moods to sleep to water retention to weight, etc. Fat in the body stores excess estrogen, making weight more difficult to lose and wreaking havoc on your moods, sleep, and more. Excess estrogen can contribute to gynecomastia in men. I recommend avoiding and eliminating soy and all soy products from your diet as much as possible. It's difficult because soy is a cheap, subsidized ingredient used in processed foods in the form of oil, thickeners, flavor enhancers, stabilizers, preservatives, and nutritive fillers. Check the ingredients list if you're eating processed food; you're probably eating soy.

---

28    Pay now or pay later...with your health. - Unknown

- **My #1 rule is...**

## *DO the BEST YOU can. PRAY over the REST, and MOVE ON with your LIFE.*

I firmly believe...No, I *know*.... that God puts a hedge of protection around you when you must eat things that are not healthy for you IF it's out of your control. God knows your heart[29], and if you are doing your best to care for your body. I don't know anyone who's prayed for God to bless their third plate of greasy enchiladas (or the bucket of ice cream you're about to eat in the closet) with any expectation of that prayer being answered.

## JUICING is healthy. <u>FALSE</u>

Because juicing strips all the fiber from the fruits and/or vegetables you're juicing, it essentially becomes pure sugar – at least your body reacts to it the same as ingesting pure sugar. (This is also true with drinking juice from the store.) Despite the concentrated amounts of phytonutrients, as soon as you drink juice, your blood sugar spikes releasing insulin and giving you a rush of energy. Within minutes, however, your blood sugar crashes because of the lack of fiber, which helps regulate the speed of digestion and absorption, leaving you feeling weak, hungry, and with a headache.

Not to mention the waste! The fibrous pulp and skin of

---

29   Jeremiah 17:10 "I the Lord search the heart and examine the mind, to reward each person according to their conduct, according to what their deeds deserve."

the fruits and vegetables are tossed in juicing. THIS GETS EXPENSIVE!

- **BLENDING** is the way to go if you are trying to get more nutrients from fruits and vegetables into your diet. Not only do you get the sweetness from the juices, but you keep the pulp and skins (fiber) that help regulate blood sugar. Because many nutrients are in the pulp and skins of fruits and vegetables, you are *boosting* nutrition with BLENDING, *getting even more vitamins, minerals, and phytonutrients than with juicing.* In addition to boosting nutrition, you are wasting nothing, and in turn, making the most of your dollar. Waste not, want not.

## You need to go on a DETOX, a CLEANSE, or a JUICE FAST to get healthy and jump start weight loss.[30] <u>FALSE FALSE FALSE!</u>

Health food stores, magazines, and celebrities are raging about (and promoting) juice fasts, colon cleanses, detox diets and "purges" to help those looking to lose weight or kick start a healthy lifestyle. But BEWARE! These therapies aren't as healthful as they may seem, and in many cases, are downright harmful to your health and your psyche.

The idea that behind these detox therapies and cleanses is that a they help the body with detoxification, or the practice of ridding the body of toxic or harmful substances. The claim is that detoxification through these methods is necessary because the body accumulates toxins through the environment, poor eating habits, or chemicals that can cause cancer and other diseases. The body needs help

---

30  2 Corinthians 7:1b "…let us purify ourselves from everything that contaminates body and spirit, perfecting holiness out of reverence for God."

getting rid of these accumulated toxins. These therapies argue that regularly cleansing oneself of toxins reduces the risk of disease - which leads to a neutral pH, radiant hair and skin, weight loss, bullet proof immunity, improved digestion, and increased energy.

*However, our bodies don't need help with this; at least not through restrictive and often dangerous detox and cleansing "therapies." That's what our livers and kidneys are for! Healthy kidneys and livers do a great job of daily cleansing our bodies without the excessive stress caused by fasts and cleanses.*

The liver is responsible for regulating, synthesizing, storing and secreting many important proteins and nutrients to the body. The liver and kidneys also purify, breakdown, and process out of the body all toxic, unwanted, or unnecessary substances that you breathe in or swallow. By turning potentially harmful "toxins" into water-soluble chemicals, healthy individuals sweat and excrete them from their bodies naturally.

**SIDE BAR:** Those who do not have healthy livers due to certain liver conditions like Hepatitis A, B, or C, alcohol-induced liver disease, or fatty liver can *possibly* accumulate toxins in their bodies. However, there is no scientific evidence that detox diets or liver cleanses help treat liver disease.

*What is a toxin?*

Anything you consume or breathe that is not a nutrient for the health of your body is a toxin (poison); natural or manmade. Air pollutants, alcohol, drugs, medicines, chemicals, nicotine, E-coli, Salmonella, etc. are all toxins; so is the metabolic waste produced by cells inside the human body. You accumulate both natural and manmade toxins when you eat or drink, and when you breathe (air pollutants). These are by-products of living in a polluted world.

However, doing a restrictive fast, cleanse, or drinking a special juice concoction or tea will not help rid your body of these toxins any faster or more effectively, according to research at Columbia University in New York.

*WHY?* Because the body is well equipped to rid itself of toxins. The liver of healthy individuals is not a place where toxins are stored.

**WAIT. READ THAT AGAIN!**

Because the LIVER DOES NOT STORE TOXINS,
detoxification products claiming to "cleanse"
the liver are USELESS.
*HMMMM.*

You would be wise to ignore – and not waste your money on - any products that make such claims, saving yourself from the restrictive and harmful effects of such "therapies."

Colon cleanses, fasting, juicing, drinking an herbal solution or eating a raw diet, are other detox therapies that have no merit and cannot live up to their claims of "healing," "rejuvenating," or "balancing" the body.

In fact, no studies have shown that juices, herbs or fasts are effective at *pulling* toxins from the blood or organs, either. Stripping nutrients and fiber (with juicing and herbal teas/remedies) along with highly restricting calories through fasting, extreme dieting, cleanses, detoxes, and "therapies" kill the healthy microflora (good gut bacteria) in the colon, wreaking havoc on your digestive system.

**What fasts, detoxes, cleanses, diets, and "therapies" can do is cause:**

- Nausea

- Vomiting

- Diarrhea

- Dramatic loss of electrolytes

- Dehydration

- Loss of nutrients (malnourishment)

- Serious medical conditions like kidney or liver failure

- Risk for possibly developing an eating disorder, and more

**SIDE BAR:** Certain carbohydrates and fats *BIND* (stick) to toxins and *HELP* flush them out of the body through waste elimination. So, to eliminate them - as a fast, detox or cleanse would have you do - would make it more difficult to rid your body of any accumulated toxins.

By now you have guessed that I do not support these radical diets or "therapies." Ultimately, *THE BENEFIT MUST OUT WEIGH THE RISK,* and there must be an actual benefit. With this in mind, there *is* a healthy and VERY beneficial plan that I do recommend: the "GUT HEALING DIET." This plan focuses on letting your digestive system heal by eating and drinking *balanced* meals that are easily digested, without overly restricting calories and giving your body the nutrients it needs.

**THE "GUT HEALING DIET" WILL:**

- reduce inflammation, bloating, and gas throughout the digestive system
- eliminate undigested food
- relieve constipation
- flood your body with the vitamins, minerals and nutrients
- eliminate indigestion, IBS, and fatigue
- help with allergies and skin issues
- reduce inflammation throughout the body

This is a great "diet" to do after vacation, the holidays, surgery or illness. I do NOT recommend doing this plan more than the suggested five days or more than two to three times a year.

**DO NOT ATTEMPT THIS "GUT HEALING DIET" IF:**

- you struggle with low weight
- you struggle or have struggled with eating disorders
- you are pregnant or trying to get pregnant
- you are nursing
- you are under the age of 18

*You can find the*
**"GUT HEALING DIET"**
*on my website at* www.getfitwithkimtoday.com.

# WHAT CRAVINGS MEAN AND HOW TO DEAL WITH THEM

We talked about how drinking water can possibly help with hunger and cravings *if you are in fact dehydrated.* However, if you're NOT dehydrated, then you can potentially become *over-hydrated* by constantly drinking water in attempts to *curb your appetite* causing more cravings and hunger pangs. Over-hydrating (drinking too much water) will flush out your electrolytes, primarily sodium. (Sodium is important for proper heart function. You cannot live without it!) When your body needs more sodium, your brain will send the hunger signal - through cravings - so you will eat something salty.

## ELECTROLYTES

You can lose electrolytes many ways. Sweating profusely from heavy exercise, working in extreme heat conditions, steam baths, saunas, and fever can all cause you to sweat out your electrolytes. Vomiting and diarrhea can lead to electrolyte loss. Certain medications, whether they are prescription or over-the-counter, can also affect your hydration levels and, in turn, electrolyte balance. Hormones greatly affect electrolytes. Genetics also play a role in whether you tend to "run low" on certain electrolytes. And finally, just drinking too much water can flush out your electrolytes. So, I'll say this again....

**Having an electrolyte imbalance can cause HUNGER.** Your brain sends signals *through cravings* to eat foods containing those missing electrolytes to get you back in balance.

**What are electrolytes?**

Electrolytes are certain nutrients within the body that perform a myriad of activities like regulating heartbeat, maintaining muscle and nerve functions, stabilizing cell walls, moving water and fluids within the body, generating energy, influencing immunity, and many other important functions.

The major electrolytes in the body are:

- Calcium

- Potassium

- Magnesium

- Sodium

- Phosphate

- Chloride

**NOTE:** Because nutrition is such a vast topic, I am only going to barely scratch the surface here. The information in this section will help give you an idea of what is *possibly* causing your cravings and hunger, and give you a few suggestions on how to handle them. Being deficient in certain electrolytes causes specific cravings. Figuring out if an electrolyte imbalance is the culprit for your cravings, hunger, and possible dehydration, is a complicated task. Blood work can assist in this area. A Certified Nutrition Specialist who specializes in Functional Nutrition, will be able to identify what is nutritionally lacking and design a program to get your body the nutrients it needs, subsequently killing your cravings. *Tackling this on your own can be overwhelming and very frustrating.*

IF YOU ARE FIGHTING INTENSE CRAVINGS, **THE FIRST STEP** IS TO IDENTIFY THE CAUSE.

**Are you truly hungry? Or....**

- Did a Dairy Queen commercial just come on TV for your favorite blizzard?

CAUSE: *SUBLIMINAL SUGGESTION or BOREDOM.*

- Did your boss just call you with more work to finish, on top of what you couldn't finish already?

CAUSE: *STRESS*

- Did you get into an argument with your spouse and are upset, angry, or have your feelings hurt?[31]

CAUSE: *EMOTION*

  ○ You *seek comfort* from an emotional response or stress through food.

- Have you not eaten for several hours (5+)?

CAUSE: *LOW BLOOD SUGAR*

  ○ If you have not eaten for several hours, your body will send the signal to eat in the form of cravings for sugar, i.e. sweets, snack foods, or fruit. Your body recognizes "sugar" (glucose) as a quick energy source. Therefore, your cravings for sweet foods are coming from your body's recognition that it needs energy, because you have not eaten in several hours. Unfortunately, your brain is not specific in the food choices. It only sends cravings for sweet tasting foods, knowing that it will get an immediate energy rush. Your body will never send you a craving for salmon, broccoli, or any specific

---

31   "For every minute you remain angry, you give up 60 seconds of peace of mind." – Ralph Waldo Emerson

"healthy" food. The brain only signals you to eat fatty, salty or sweet foods. This unfortunately translates into chocolate, candy, chips, pretzels, cookies, energy drinks, coffee, etc. for most of us.

Determining the **CAUSE** of your cravings may be a difficult task and involve some self-examining.

**However, this is KEY INFORMATION for you because:**

- If you are DEHYDRATED for any reason, then drinking water *will help* with your hunger and cravings. Remember that "thirst" feels like "hunger." Because many fresh foods like fruits and vegetables have a high-water content, your body may confuse the desire to *eat* those foods to get the necessary hydration, when in fact, your body *needs* WATER, not food. However, if the only reason you crave a blizzard is because you just saw the advertisement on TV, then you can rest assured that your craving was a subconscious trigger to your brain for a sweet treat. As much as we might wish it true, your body will never *need* a blizzard. In this case, distract yourself! Go outside and walk 10-15 minutes. Or turn off the TV!

- If it's an *EMOTIONAL response to a STRESSFUL situation,* then you can implement *self-control* and decide how you're going to proceed.[32] Are you going to indulge and try to gain comfort from food? Or are you going to pick a healthier direction by getting your comfort from resolving the conflict?

- If you STRESS EAT when faced with an overwhelming task

---

32    Hebrews 4:15 "For we do not have a high priest who is unable to empathize with our weaknesses, but we have one who has been tempted in every way, just as we are - yet he did not sin."

or deadline, then you may need to implement or learn time management skills; ask for help (you'd be amazed at how much people will help you if you only ask); or take a few deep breaths, put your head down, and suck it up buttercup. Do the best you can.

- And finally, if you have *NOT EATEN in several hours,* then eat and fuel your body. Again, you have the choice to pick foods that you know your body needs. Ultimately, even though your brain sends a craving for "sugar," you are always in control of what you put in your mouth, even if you may not *feel* like it at the time.

Once you have identified the CAUSE of your HUNGER and CRAVINGS, then you can SUCCESSFULLY STOP any bad habit, and instead give your body the nutrients and/or water it *NEEDS.*

This is where WILLPOWER comes in and you make a choice:

*Are you going to give in to that craving?*

**Or**

*Are you going to use the knowledge that you've gained in this book[33] and choose water, fish, rice, potatoes, chicken, vegetables, soup, or fruit over cookies, candy, chips, hamburgers, fries, soda, energy drinks, etc.?*

**Once you realize where the craving is coming from YOU have the POWER, the SELF-CONTROL, and the CHOICEto change the direction of your health.**

---

33   James 3:13 "Who is wise and understanding among you? Let him show it by his good life, by deeds done in the humility that comes from wisdom."

## WILLPOWER and Temptation

Do you have it? Do you think everyone except you seems to have it? Would you pay any amount for it? What if I told you nobody *automatically* has willpower, but we *all* can get it?

Look at this scenario:

*Word of the day.... WILLPOWER.*

*It's been one of those weeks (or 2) where good intentions and plans get tossed out the window by 10:00 am. I planned on working out this morning as usual, but nope. It didn't happen. By the time I stopped and looked at the clock, it was 6pm! WHAT?!? Now, I need to get supper on the table. I'm frustrated, exhausted, it's cold outside, and I DO NOT want to go to the gym and fight the crowd. I can feel my anxiety creeping in as my face flushes and negative thoughts surface. Yes, I love to work out, but I am **struggling** with the "I don't want to's." BIG TIME!*

Can you relate?

I can, because this is literally an excerpt from my *personal journal on January 21, 2014!*

Flashback to the rest of that entry....

*This brings me back to the word of the day.... WILLPOWER. This is a funny word to me. It's very deceiving in a way, because it can bring positive thoughts when you have it, and negative, destructive thoughts when you don't. WILLPOWER— It comes. It goes. And you never know when, where, or why it may or may not grace you with its presence.*

*I have the WILL – to workout, get fit, eat right, be healthy, yada yada yada - but from time to time (like tonight), the POWER is missing. That's when friends and my support system are crucial.[34] Tracy was there to encourage me and give me a swift kick out the door. And, of course, I got a great workout. I feel better, and my mood improved. And the best part? I ended the day with a feeling of success and accomplishment towards my goals instead of a defeated spirit. It's funny how just one hour can change the outlook on your entire day!*

One of the most common statements I hear people make when talking with me about their diet is "I just don't have any willpower. I can't pass up ----fill in the blank----." WILLPOWER is thought of as this magical trait we admire in others and see the lack of as a flaw in ourselves. **However, that's just not true!**

We justify our actions by allowing ourselves to be *victims of WILLPOWER.* We need to take control of our choices and OWN them. Let's start by realizing that we *do* have control over what we put in our mouths, what we say, what we do, and how we react. We all struggle with some form of self-control in our lives, but the fact is....

*We DO have the ability to strengthen our willpower in any area of our lives.*

**THE FIRST STEP TO STRENGTHENING YOUR WILLPOWER:**

Accepting the fact that we all have the "WILL" but not always the "POWER." The Bible states that "The spirit is willing, but the body is weak." Matthew 26:41b.

---

34 Proverbs 27:17 "As iron sharpens iron, so one man sharpens another."

I believe most of us truly want to change, but feel powerless to do so, because we don't know how. Our bad habits seem to be too ingrained in us.[35] There is hope! **Self-control is a gift that we already possess**, and we can hire people to teach us what we don't know (like with diet and exercise).

*"But the fruit of the Spirit is love, joy, peace, patience, kindness, goodness, faithfulness, gentleness, and self-control."*
*Galatians 5:22-23a*

**THE NEXT STEP:**

Take control of what you can control.

We are all faced with temptation. Our misconception is that we must *fight* it. I think we can agree that it's futile to try and fight temptation. Whatever you focus on grows–good and bad!

**Since we can't fight temptation, "RUN, FORREST! RUN!"**
(to take a quote from the movie "Forrest Gump").

You can flee from temptation. If there are certain places, people, or activities that tempt you to eat sweets (for example), then stay away from those people, places and activities. Some people can bring you down easier than you can bring them up. You may have to separate yourself from them for a while, or forever. [36]

---

35   Let your faith be bigger than your fear. - Unknown

36   1 Corinthians 15:33 "Do not be misled: 'Bad company corrupts good character.'"

**THE FINAL STEP:**

Own it!

Let's be honest. We know when we are about to make a bad choice. None of us *unknowingly* eat all the Halloween candy before the trick-or-treaters come. So, a great way to gain some of your "POWER" back, is by saying *"I don't* (or won't) pass up the Halloween candy" instead of saying *"I can't* pass up the Halloween candy." By owning your choice, good or bad, it puts *you in CONTROL.* (Of course, with control and choice comes greater responsibility and consequences.) Hopefully, that is liberating news for you!

By *choosing* to not give in to your cravings, to not look to food, or even exercise for comfort, to gain control of your POWER through self-control and good choices—you will create healthy habits that will become a way of life. If you STOP in the middle of the downward spiral and PRAY[37] through it, making good choices will become easier. [38]

**WILLPOWER** is a chain reaction that starts by making one good choice, and they add up quickly! Baby steps will lead to small victories. Those victories turn into giant gains, which translate into success,[39] but you must be deliberate in your actions and choices. Instead of focusing on what you *don't want* to do,

---

37   Ephesians 3:20 "Now to Him who is able to do immeasurably more than all we ask or imagine, according to His power that is at work within us."

38   We become what we repeatedly do. Excellence, therefore, is not an act, but a habit. - Aristotle

39   Achieve success in any area of life by identifying the optimum strategies and repeating them until they become habits. – Charles J. Givens

focus on what you *do want* to do. And encourage others to do the same.

When the world is weighing you down, and you don't know what to do; grab the "WILL" you do have. Call someone who can help you get the "POWER," and go workout or step away from the cookie! Just remember that God's always on speed dial, but sometimes He comes in the form of a good friend (or a mean personal trainer. Ha-ha!)

## MY STORY:

I have personally struggled with binge eating episodes periodically throughout my adult life. Whatever contributes to the "episode," I now know that if I get a handle on it *immediately*, it will not grip me for very long. It's momentary. However, this took *years* of practice and prayer to learn. I am not naïve enough to think that my struggles with food, or my inclination to turn to food for comfort in times of stress, disappointment, and anxiety, are over. Realizing that I may struggle this way to some degree helps me stay diligent in prayer, dependent on God for my strength[40], and keeps me humble.

I specifically remember a few years ago, when I literally said, "I have totally figured out how to keep weight off. I know exactly what works." Oh, was I ever wrong! It was not long after – weeks actually – that I became extremely ill, going on the worst health "ride" of my life. Consequently, gaining 40 lbs. in the process, despite my "perfect

---

40    Psalm 71:16 "I will walk in the strength of the Lord. I will tell everyone that You alone are just and good."

epiphany diet plan." I didn't even realize at the time how pride had crept into my life.

I could totally relate to Paul when he wrote about his struggle to do what he knows is right. He's tormented by the fact that he continues to do what he hates, despite the fact he knows it's wrong, bad for him, and he doesn't *want* to do it. He writes that he is "like a slave to his sin." Later, he comes to understand that he is not a slave to it any longer. I encourage you to read his words in Romans 7:7 – 8:39.

In another passage (2 Corinthians 12:1-10), Paul goes on to explain how he prayed and prayed for God to take the "thorn" from his side. And how he realized, finally, that his strength came from the fact he would never be free from the "thorn" because it kept him from becoming conceited. Paul recognized that through his struggle, he became more reliant on God for his strength and power. The "thorn" helped him be dependent on God instead of himself. Not only did this [reliance on God] make Paul better, but also made him joyful, content, and happy.

**SIDE BAR:** There are many theories as to what Paul's "thorn" was. I'm not sure it even matters to me other than sheer curiosity. Maybe his "thorn" was left vague so that more people could relate to him and his torment. The point is we all have a "thorn" – whether physical, emotional, or mental – that weakens us. Until we see that in our weakness we become strong because of the necessity for us to rely on God, we will resent and fight against our "thorn."[41] Whatever it is.

---

41 Proverbs 11:2 "When pride comes, then comes disgrace, but with humility comes wisdom."

It took me several years, but I can say that I, too, am thankful for my struggles.[42] This has not always been the case, and there are those hard days I wish I didn't struggle with food. BUT, they are few and far between because I realize God has gifted me in the very area that I struggle with most.

I know He has done this for three reasons:

1)  I will stay humble and dependent on Him, alone.
2)  I will find my worth in Him and not in my appearance or abilities;
3)  And most importantly, so I can help others, give them hope, and lead them to Him.

I realize if God took away my "thorn" then my passion for fitness, nutrition, cooking, and helping others through the emotional battlegrounds of food addiction would also leave me. In turn, this book would never have been written. I couldn't be there for you.

Today, if God gave me the choice to take away my struggle - knowing all of that - I would say, "No." There is no way I would trade a second, a lesson, a friendship, or an opportunity that He has given me through my hardships and struggles.

By allowing us to struggle and resist our temptations, God is making us stronger against them. Temptations begin to have less and less of a hold over us every time we successfully resist them, and instead be obedient to God. The

---

42   Psalm 119: 71 "It was good for me to be afflicted so that I might learn your decrees."

temptation may never completely go away, but with His strength, it will become easier to resist.

> **SIDE BAR:** If you are struggling with self-worth issues...
>
> Know that You were ESPECIALLY made...ON PURPOSE... for a REASON...with LOVE, by LOVE, and for LOVE. "....GOD IS LOVE." 1 John 4:8b
>
> I encourage you to read Psalm 139:13-16. I almost wrote the verses out for you here, but there is something powerfully moving about looking them up yourself and reading them directly from the Bible, OUT LOUD.

Learn to look at every struggle as an opportunity to grow, improve, and help somebody else.[43] You can help someone in your time of need by allowing them to reap the blessing from helping you.[44] You see, even when you're the one reaching up for a hand, the person reaching down to help you up is also being blessed. At some point, the tables will turn, and you will reach down to pull someone else up out of their pit—reaping the harvest of blessings from your act.[45]

---

43　Doing nothing for others is the undoing of ourselves. – Horace Mann

44　Proverbs 11:25 "A generous man will prosper; he who refreshes others will himself be refreshed."

45　Philippians 2:3-4 "Do nothing out of selfish ambition or vain conceit. Rather, in humility value others above yourselves, not looking to your own interests but each of you to the interests of the others."

**If you feel the need to turn to food for comfort from stress or anxiety**:

➢ Pray for strength, comfort, self-control, peace, calm, a healthy distraction, etc. to avoid a potential binge eating episode. In fact, *Pray Through Everything:* hard times, good times, before you eat, before getting up; before working out, during your workout, after your workout, at work, while you play, while you rest, before and during conversations, and in your relationships.[46]

➢ Be *INTENTIONAL* in your actions, your plans, and your prayers. Then, get dressed in "real" clothes (not stretchy sweatpants or yoga pants), and leave the house – i.e. the temptation. This may be the "out" God is providing you.

*"No temptation has overtaken you except what is common to mankind. And God is faithful; He will not let you be tempted beyond what you can bear. But when you are tempted, He will also provide a way out so that you can endure it." 1 Corinthians 10:13.*

## WEIGHT LOSS SURGERY – Yea or Nay?

I have been a certified expert in the nutrition and fitness fields for over 26 years.

- Personal Trainer
- Triathlon Coach
- Group Aerobics Instructor

---

46    1 Thessalonians 5:16-18 "Rejoice always, pray continually, give thanks in all circumstances; for this is God's will for you in Christ Jesus."

- Aerobics Instructor Trainer
- Fitness Nutrition Specialist
- Youth Exercise Specialist
- Senior Exercise Specialist
- Positional Isometrics Coach
- Rossiter Coach
- CrossFit Endurance Coach
- And many more subcategories

I have lived and breathed what I write and teach to my clients and others in this book and through my business. *So, how do I feel about weight loss surgery?*

## I AM <u>NOT</u> AGAINST WEIGHT LOSS SURGERY.

Yes, you read that right.

It may surprise you, but I am not opposed to weight loss surgery...

*IF* it's done the right way
*AND* for the right reasons.

Let me explain....

There is no doubt that food has emotional and psychological aspects, and for some people it's a strong-hold that they cannot control or break free from on their own. It's been proven that certain foods help the brain release feel-good chemicals like serotonin when eaten. Science has even speculated that some foods (like sugar, bread, caffeine, chocolate, dairy, etc.) have an addictive quality to them, much like heroin. When a person stops eating those addictive foods, they do experience withdrawal symptoms which drastically affect emotions and mood, making lifestyle changes even more difficult.

People experience emotions like those felt after losing a loved one - depression, guilt, and even grief - when attempting to give up certain foods and drinks, drugs, cigarettes, and alcohol. I have had clients tell me they rely on food for comfort, strength, confidence, etc. Of course, they also feel the repercussions of transferring their "POWER" to food – guilt, shame, failure, judgement.

For weight loss surgery patients to not address the psychological and emotional ties they have with food is setting them up to fail, gain the weight back— plus more—and potentially cause serious *irreversible* damage to their bodies.

That being said, I do believe there are some very specific instances where weight loss surgery can be life changing and very healthy for some individuals. For me to support the surgery there are definite criteria to be met.

1) Are you more than 100 lbs. overweight?
2) Has your doctor advised you to lose more than 150 lbs. for health reasons?
3) Have you exercised *consistently and daily* for at least one year?
4) Have you hired a fitness professional to structure a *focused* exercise program *specifically* for you?
5) Have you made significant and healthy nutritional changes to your diet?

6) Have you been *consistent* with healthy nutritional diet changes for at least one year?

7) Have you hired a nutrition professional to structure a *focused* nutrition program *specifically* for you?

8) Have you sought emotional help with your ties to food? (This could be through professional psychological therapy and/or counseling, spiritual counseling and Biblical studies.) Have you continued with this therapy for at least one year?

9) Do you have a strong support system in place?

10) Have you put in place healthy lifestyle changes, and implemented and practiced those changes for at least one year?

I do not see weight loss surgery as a viable option for those who *do not* answer *Yes* to the above questions. Weight loss surgery should be used as a TOOL, along with lifestyle changes in exercise, nutrition, and the psychological and emotional relationships with others, food, and oneself.

*Weight loss surgery can be that little extra help to allow the change needed for a healthy life.* If done correctly, weight loss surgery can mean the difference between life and death, in many ways.

## BACK TO BASICS

There are some very basic truths to remember when trying to adopt or adapt a healthy lifestyle and wade through all the information available. When you start to feel overwhelmed, review these BASIC TRUTHS:

1) **Eat when you're hungry. Stop eating when you're full.** Do not eat a certain amount because it's "what you're supposed to do" according to the latest trend. If you are *not* hungry, then *don't eat!* Now that being said, don't starve yourself either. Going long periods of time (more than 24 hours) without eating will kill your appetite and stop your metabolism from working efficiently—potentially developing into an eating disorder. Eating triggers your hunger mechanism and kick starts your metabolism.

2) Eating "healthy" food, doing cleanses, and exercising like a maniac to offset poor nutrition will not do anything for weight loss. **The key is** finding a way to eat fewer *total* calories, while getting all the nutrition (micronutrients, macronutrients, and water) needed. Exercise keeps your body strong and healthy for LIVING. Weight loss is a side benefit of exercise, *BUT exercise does not = weight loss!*

   As you learn *your* body, you will know *when* and *how much* to eat to maintain your perfect weight and health. Everyone is different and needs to learn what works best for *their* body. This is where your food JOURNAL plays a key role in your weight management and overall health.

3) The human body was designed to **MOVE. Period.** Our bodies, even if broken, need physical activity *every day*

- for most of the day - to function properly on the inside and outside. We are a living organism that is constantly using muscle contractions to keep us alive. There is truth to the phrase "move it or lose it." Muscles will atrophy if they are not being used.

If you are suffering from:

- chronic pain (arthritis, fibromyalgia, restless leg syndrome, cramps, tendonitis)
- digestive issues
- bowel issues
- insomnia
- hormone issues (thyroid, menopause, metabolic syndrome)
- brain issues (depression, anxiety, poor memory)
- disease (cancer, diabetes, insulin resistance, heart)
- skeletal and nerve issues (bone density, chronic misalignments, sciatica)

Moving *more* will significantly help and possibly cure many of these ailments. And you don't necessarily have to run marathons or flip tractor tires to do it! The fact is, we are not moving enough. If you are not moving much of the day, your body is not going to be able to function or digest the food you eat properly. If you are not digesting your food properly, then you cannot get the nutrients you need to be healthy and function well.

4) The human body was designed to **digest Food** to get the proper nutrients it needs in the proper amounts and combinations – *not* protein bars and shakes, boxed and

packaged meals, or pills and supplements. Liquid diets, restrictive food group and elimination diets (unless you have a diagnosed allergy or severe sensitivity to specific foods), and calorie and macronutrient restrictive diets will only cause you problems down the road.

These restrictions can lead to the development of:

- disease
- illnesses (low immunity, malnourishment)
- weight gain (metabolic disorders)
- musculoskeletal disorders/problems (insufficient macronutrients = carbs, protein, fats)

If you aren't getting enough protein, carbohydrates and fats in proper ratios, then you *will not* be able to heal and recover from exercise or injury properly. Also, if you are not eating a wide variety of colorful foods (fruits and veggies) you *will not* be able to get enough vitamins, minerals, fiber, and water in the proper ratios. Yes, I hear some of you saying, "That's what vitamins and protein shakes are for!" True, but let's face facts, man-made is never going to be as good for you as God-made.

While there are situations that require "supplementation," the meaning of the term "SUPPLEMENT" is: *in addition to. NOT in place of.*

While I'm not at all advocating eliminating necessary medications or vitamins where there is a diagnosed deficiency, I do think we can agree that human beings need to EAT and CHEW actual food to maintain optimal health; which leads me into the next point.

5) **Chew** your food thoroughly. Rushing through meals leads to overeating and does nothing for your digestive system. If you are not properly digesting your food (which starts in the mouth), then you cannot get all the nutrients.

Undigested food leads to gas, bloating, indigestion, constipation, etc., which leads to diseases and weight gain. "Use it or lose it," also applies here. If you are not chewing food (liquid diets), your digestive system will become "sluggish" not allowing food to move through the intestines and out the body. This can lead to leaky gut syndrome and constipation. Liquid diets do not provide a sustainable number of calories and are typically deficient in carbs, protein, or fat. Most who try long term liquid diets for weight loss risk becoming malnourished and regain any weight lost.

6) **Size matters.** Overeating wreaks havoc on your digestive system and your waistline. It doesn't matter if you are overeating "healthy" food, either. Eating the proper PORTIONS matters with *all* foods. Your body is only capable of digesting and using a certain amount of food at a time. Overworking your organs will eventually lead to back-up and problems sooner than later. If you regularly suffer from indigestion, gas, bloating, or acid reflux, you may be overeating.

7) **Hydrate properly.** The human body must have water to be able to digest food, lubricate joints and soft tissues, transport nutrients, and remove waste and toxins from the body. Water is best, but if you struggle with drinking throughout the day, try incorporating hydrating foods into your diet. My trick is eating vegetable soups (I get my

vitamins and minerals here, too!), melons, cucumbers, green smoothies (more vitamins and minerals!!), and herbal teas. But nothing is as good as plain ole' water.

8) **Catch some RAYS and more ZZZZ's.** Sunshine and sleep go hand in hand. Most of us sit inside all day. If we don't get enough sunshine (15-20 minutes a day of direct sunlight), then our bodies don't get proper usable amounts of vitamin D (for bone health) and cannot produce proper amounts of the sleep hormone, melatonin. Without the production of melatonin, our sleep suffers.

> **TIP:** If you will walk 15-20 minutes after lunch or work, you can aid digestion, get your rays, and a little extra exercise at the same time. Better yet, do your workout outside!

9) **Be your own advocate.** Much of what I teach clients is how to read their bodies: which foods digests well; what hunger feels like; what fullness feels like; the difference between muscle soreness, fatigue, injury, tiredness, and just lack of motivation; what feeling *good* actually feels like! Most people I work with don't remember what it feels like to have energy and *feel good*.

The one thing I impress upon them and repeat over and over is:

You are living in that body – no one else. Only *you* know how certain things feel. If something is not working, even if it's "supposed" to be working, then speak up! Everyone is different in their body chemistry and not every medication, food, exercise, supplement, etc. works well for everyone.

10) **Be PATIENT.** The idea of having patience for weight loss is frustrating because we all want the weight to be gone yesterday, but there is only so much you can do in one day. *You didn't get in the shape you're in now overnight.* So, it stands to reason that your body will not heal and transform overnight either. There is a limit to how hard we can push our bodies. If you try to push too hard, injury and rebound weight gain will be the result. Accept the pace that your body heals, gets in shape, and loses weight. Everyone is different.

To be successful, approach weight loss with the mindset of balance by staying positive, rewarding yourself for small successes, cutting yourself some slack and forgiving yourself for slip-ups. Have patience through the process. This will lead to PERMANENT weight loss, LIFE-LONG health, and EASIER weight management.

Losing weight and getting in shape takes effort, but it shouldn't take over your life. It only feels that way when you try to do too much too fast. You should still have the ability and freedom to enjoy social events and eat foods you love in moderation, while maintaining a healthy weight. Patience is a virtue we can all use more liberally.

## KEEPING A HEALTHY PERSPECTIVE

I personally have done it ALL in efforts to stay on track nutritionally at parties, functions, events, vacations, and even holidays:

- Don't eat
- Take my own food
- Partake with no food restrictions

These strategies have their place and work in different circumstances, but before you decide to implement any of them, ask yourself:

- Why am I doing this?
- Is it going to cause someone else to stumble and fall off their "wagon?"

  Read Romans 14.

- Is it going to hurt someone's feelings?
- Is it really going to help or hinder my health goals?

If you feel like you're living an isolated and highly restrictive life to lose weight, then you're likely being too restrictive. You will eventually burn out if this is the case.

The best advice I can offer is to *be mindful* of what you are eating, *pray* over it, *be thankful,* and *do the best you can.* One meal is not going to make or break you if you are living out a healthy lifestyle *every* day.

**If it's made *especially* for you with *love,* then God *will bless it* and the calories don't count if you eat a little!**

Your lifestyle is made up of your habits, and your habits are made up of what you do every day. If you want to live a healthy and happy lifestyle, look at what you *consistently* do daily. Then take the necessary steps to change anything that does not fit into *your* definition of a HEALTHY and HAPPY LIFESTYLE.

# SUN & SUPPLEMENTS

I believe most people can get all the nutrients they need by eating a well-balanced diet. However, sometimes your body may get off-track for various reasons and needs a little help getting back on track. That's what **SUPPLEMENTATION** is for – *a tool used to help you fill in the gaps when diet alone cannot meet all your needs.*

## WHAT IS A SUPPLEMENT?

The definition of a supplement is: *In addition to; Extra; Something that completes, enhances, or adds to something else.* Note that it does not say *"Replaces" or "Instead of."*

Supplements should be just that – supplemental – used in addition to good nutrition. They are not to be used *in place of* food. This is where people get confused. Many people try to use a pill form of a nutrient to replace eating a well-balanced diet.

The only reasons supplements should *replace* food is if the individual:

1) has an allergy to specific foods – like suffering from Celiac Disease.

2) has other limiting factors that require supplementation – like living in places (Alaska or Seattle for example) with limited sunlight (Vitamin D).

3) cannot digest a specific food – like having their gall bladder removed.

4) has been prescribed a supplement for other medical reasons.

Don't get too bogged down with supplements. Terms like HGH,

DHEA, Macro Ratios, Essential Oils, Probiotics, Prebiotics (not to mention all the herbs, vitamins, minerals) lead to confusion, frustration, and a cabinet full of pills. If you take more supplements than you are eating nutritious foods and exercising consistently, it's time to reevaluate your program.

## ARE SUPPLEMENTS NECESSARY?

You can only know for certain if you have a deficiency in a vitamin, mineral, or hormone if you have your blood and urine tested. Those tests provide a clear picture of deficiencies. If it's not possible to "fix" these issues with diet and exercise alone, then take supplements with the guidance of your doctor and nutritionist. Be sure to continue eating and exercising to *support* the benefits of those supplements.

Supplements should never be taken in place of eating a nutritious, balanced diet, *unless* you have specific reasons that inhibit you from getting those necessary nutrients from food.

*Supplements are a TOOL used to help get the nutrients you need for a short period of time, with the intension of ultimately meeting those needs nutritionally through your diet.*

### WHEN TO TAKE SUPPLEMENTS

- You are sick.
- You are recovering from illness, injury, surgery, or cancer treatments.
- You have a known/diagnosed deficiency.

- You are training for an ultra-endurance sport/event (triathlon, marathon, soccer).

- You must limit or eliminate certain foods due to a food allergy or intolerance – recommended by a doctor.

- You are taking medications that require certain vitamins/minerals be supplemented due to restrictions of certain foods or food groups.

- The elderly, who don't or cannot eat enough variety or calories, should take supplements recommended by their doctors.

- You are dealing with a high level of ACUTE stress (new job, death, divorce, getting married, moving, holidays, etc.). ACUTE stress is short-term.

**NOTE:** Supplements can be taken while dealing with CHRONIC stress, but sooner or later the chronic stress *must* be resolved to avoid long-term physical effects.

## HOW TO TAKE SUPPLEMENTS

I highly recommend the practice of CYCLING on and off supplements, *unless* you have a medical reason to remain on a supplement for an extended period.

**NOTE:** If tests reveal a nutrient deficiency, plan to get retested every 2-3 months until your levels are in a normal range. This determines how long to take a specified supplement.

Cycling assures you do not get too much of a nutrient. Too much of a nutrient can do as much, and sometimes more, harm than too little. For example, taking too much Omega-3 Fatty Acids can potentially increase your risk for developing prostate cancer; too much iron can block other minerals and vitamins from being absorbed by the body.

Watch for food products being "fortified" with nutrients such as calcium, vitamin D, and Omega-3 Fatty Acids. If you take supplements *and* eat "fortified" foods, you run the risk of potentially over-dosing on some nutrients.

Getting too much of a "good thing" (nutrient) is a cumulative process. This is another reason I recommend cycling on and off supplements *and* foods.

*Supplement cycles are generally 6-12 weeks depending on the supplement, current health status, and level of physical activity.*

Different supplements can require different doses, combinations, and timing to work properly. This is where a Certified Nutritionist specializing in Functional Medicine and Nutrition can be an asset to you. You will *save money* in the long run because they guide you in exactly what you need and how to effectively take it. Otherwise, you are wasting your money and not getting the desired benefits and results from supplements.

**Other items besides "pills" fall into the SUPPLEMENT category:**

- Meal replacement drinks/shakes/smoothies
- Meal replacement powders
- Meal replacement bars

- Protein powders

- Protein bars

- Protein drinks/shakes/smoothies

These should also be used to help *fill in the gaps* of your nutrition profile (diet) when you either *cannot* eat a proper meal due to scheduling or travel, OR because you need additional nutrients you can't get from food alone.

I call shakes, powders, and bars "Emergency Foods" because they should *not* be a STAPLE in your diet.

It is crucial to choose these items wisely because they are typically full of:

- Sugar

- Artificial sweeteners

- Chemicals

- Fillers

- Soy – acts as an estrogen in the body (both male and female; adult and child) and is one of the most genetically modified (GMO) foods on the planet.

- Whey – not an easily digestible form of protein causing gas, bloating, and other digestive issues.

- Casein – milk based protein with the same effects as whey.

- Other ingredients that are either not easily digestible (causing gas, bloating, or constipation) and/or potentially interact with other medications and supplements you may be taking.

- Fat and calories.

In some cases, I've found that specific protein powders, supplements, bars, and shakes can help jump-start my clients' nutrition in the beginning phases of their specific program.

## Here is a brief OVERVIEW of a few supplements I recommend in both Food and Pill form:

**Note:** *This is not a complete or detailed list. Doses are determined in conjunction with a client's blood work and prescriptions on a case-by-case basis.*

**OMEGA-3 Fatty Acids:**

Reduce inflammation in the body; good for heart health, joints, and brain health

- FOOD: wild caught fatty fish (salmon, tuna, mackerel), milled flax seed, Chia seeds (in the form of gel or ground), Cacao.
- PILL: *only if a client cannot or will not eat the food sources*

It must:

- Contain 500 EPA / 250 DHA
- Be Molecularly Distilled
- Be Enteric Coated (This keeps you from being the "stinky" kid in class!)

## VITAMIN D:

Responsible for increasing the intestinal absorption of calcium and other minerals.

- In the form of direct, daily SUNSHINE. [47]

  There is no substitute for sunshine in your life. It's the most absorbable form of Vitamin D, it boosts moods, regulates your circadian rhythm, aids in the production of melatonin so you can sleep, and helps you appreciate the amazing creations of God. I cannot express in words the healing properties of sunshine. [48]

- I recommend 15-25 minutes of direct sunshine daily. The amount will be determined by the season and your location. West Texas sun is very hot, and the seasons are mild. Therefore, 15 minutes a day is plenty. For those living in more northern parts of the country, you may need longer exposure to get enough vitamin D from the sun. You may need to supplement Vitamin D-3 in pill form.

- If you are prone to skin cancer and are concerned with UV rays, limit the amount of unprotected sunshine to 10 minutes per day or supplement with Vitamin D-3 in pill form.

  - Try coconut oil topically as a sunscreen. Coconut oil has natural sunscreen properties and will not cause skin irritation for those with skin sensitivities. I am allergic to all sunscreens on the market. I have used

---

47  Keep your face always toward the sunshine and the shadows will fall behind you. – Walt Whitman

48  SUNSHINE JUST MAKES YOU HAPPY! – Kim Clinkenbeard

coconut oil as my personal sunscreen for decades with success. Coconut oil also provides protection from the harmful rays of the sun without blocking your body's ability to absorb vitamin D.

## MAGNESIUM

Necessary for protein synthesis, muscle and nerve function, blood glucose control, blood pressure regulation, and more.

- FOOD: This is always addressed in my clients' individual nutrition profiles. Although nuts are a great source of magnesium, I generally do NOT include nuts or nut butters in the beginning phases of a program.

- EPSOM SALT BATHS: find details and the recipe in the BEAUTY SECTION

- PILL: Under supervision and only if clients cannot get adequate amounts through food and/or Epsom Salt baths.

  It must contain Magnesium from:

  - Oxide
  - Citrate
  - Malate

## PROBIOTICS

Probiotics help populate your gut with good bacteria which is necessary for proper digestion of food, immune health, mood and brain function. Your gut (digestive system) is known as your SECOND BRAIN.

- What kills good gut bacteria?
  - A diet high in processed foods = sugar and starchy carbs

- ◦ Alcohol
- ◦ Certain medications: antibiotics, NSAIDS, aspirin, antacids
- ◦ Stress!

- What are the side effects of low gut bacteria?
  - ◦ Poor gut health
  - ◦ Little absorption of nutrients
  - ◦ Weakened immunity
  - ◦ Gas and bloating
  - ◦ Chronic inflammation and the development of inflammatory diseases, like IBS, arthritis, heart disease, and depression
  - ◦ Skin issues, and more!

**NOTE:** You can get yourself in a real pickle - no pun intended; well, maybe a little – if you take too many probiotics. Some people have an over-abundance of gut bacteria, and it will wreak havoc because you have too many of the little buggers duking it out in your tummy! Start slowly when introducing probiotics into your regimen. The best way to navigate through all of this and get the right probiotic, at the right dosages, is to work with a Certified Nutritionist specializing in Functional Medicine and Nutrition. Seek these professionals out if you have SIBO (Small Intestine Bacteria Overgrowth), yeast overgrowth, allergies, histamines, or cannot tolerate fermented foods.

- Because the body does not make probiotics (good gut bacteria), it's necessary to *feed* them. Taking probiotics does not mean you are creating or *keeping* the healthy gut bacteria if you continue to eat a poor diet that kills them off. You must feed the good gut bacteria certain foods (prebiotics) by eating a healthy diet. This keeps your gut healthy and HAPPY. Prebiotics are a form of soluble fiber.

- Foods containing prebiotics are:
  - » Garlic, onions, leeks, sweet potatoes, dandelion greens, jicama
- Probiotic FOOD sources: Fermented foods (Sauerkraut, fermented vegetables), Kombucha; NOT DAIRY PRODUCTS (even those claiming to be high in probiotics)!
- PILL: the most important factor in choosing a probiotic is that they are ALIVE. These should be purchased in the refrigerated section and contain a minimum of 30 billion CFU's (Colony-Forming Units) from *several different* strains. Beside *each strain* (not total for the bottle!) it must say *CFU*. Probiotics should be refrigerated and taken daily, AFTER you have changed your diet and healed your gut of unhealthy bacteria.

**NOTE:** If you are taking a probiotic but are unwilling to change your diet, then you are just wasting your money.

**THE MOST BENEFICIAL SUPPLEMENT for those making significant healthy nutritional changes in their diets is, by far, DIGESTIVE ENZYMES.**

- Digestive enzymes help you digest proteins, carbs, and fats more efficiently and completely. Without proper and complete digestion, you can't absorb or transport nutrients from food or supplements.

- My clients take a digestive enzyme in the very beginning stages of their nutrition program. After evaluation, they have the option to continue taking them on an "as needed" basis, dependent upon their specific food tolerances.

  ◦ Digestive enzymes should contain a blend that helps digest protein, fat, carbs, fiber, and milk sugar.

**PROTEIN POWDER**

- I recommend a plant based protein powder (particularly pea protein), because it's a more digestible form of protein. For delicate stomachs, myself included, even rice based protein powders can cause severe stomach upset and digestive issues. As with all packaged food products, look for protein powders containing *food* ingredients - no artificial flavors, sweeteners, additives, chemicals, soy, or byproducts.

  ◦ Protein powders, bars, and shakes should be used in *moderation* and not in place of whole foods. I categorize these supplements as "emergency" foods, reserved for when I travel, can't find something nutritious to eat, or find myself in a situation where I don't have time for a proper meal (like when I was waiting at the hospital for my nephew to be born).

# BEAUTY

**GUYS! THIS SECTION IS FOR YOU, TOO.** Well, minus the "makeup" discussion. Unless you use it for Halloween.

[49]I have always had very sensitive skin. I'm allergic to makeup, moisturizers, creams, makeup remover, soaps, lotions, fragrances, and sunscreen. ALL sunscreen. The first time we noticed it was when I was about 8 or 9 years old, and my parents took me and my brother on a canoeing trip. Being responsible parents, they slathered us in sunscreen for three straight days. We camped on the Rio Grande River, so there were no mirrors. I'll never forget finally getting back to civilization and seeing my reflection in the truck mirror. Oh, the horror! My face was a complete round circle. I looked like the Man in the Moon! We finally figured out it was a bad reaction to sunscreen. (The weird thing with my skin is that it may take a day, or 30, to react to a product, which was the case on that trip. You will have your own peculiarities.)

Since that episode, I tried every hypoallergenic sunscreen, soap, lotion, etc. I have still not found a moisturizer or sunscreen I can use. I've noticed that as I've gotten older, my skin has become even more sensitive. I rarely wear makeup, because after a few hours, my eyes itch like crazy! However, I have figured out skincare solutions for everything I need to take care of my skin and stay as young looking as possible.

I'm thrilled to share them with you! Even if you don't have skin sensitivities but are looking for more natural skincare products, these solutions are great for your skin, health, and budget.

---

49    Happy girls are the prettiest! – Audrey Hepburn

**SIDE BAR:** I have found some store-bought soap and lotions that work well for me, but most of my skincare is from food sources. While I do not feel right about promoting certain brand-name items in this book, I will be happy to give you those if you contact me through my website at www.getfitwithkimtoday.com. This ensures you get the most updated list as brands, businesses, and products change. Or if I find something better or cheaper.

I'm a girl who tends to be more on the lazy side of beauty regimens. So, all my tips and recipes are super easy, cheap, and make enough to freeze and use for months! There is little to no time involved in making these, and my skincare routine takes all of five minutes a day!

*Are you ready?* Here we go!

## *My personal daily face regimen*

### FIRST:

Remove eye makeup with coconut oil.

### SECOND:

Wash face using a Buf-Puf Exfoliating Facial Cleansing Sponge with goat's milk and food based soap. Scrub gently in circular motions over face and neck. Rinse with cool water.

### THIRD:

Dip a cotton pad or cotton ball into my homemade FACIAL TONER and wipe over entire face and neck. Let this dry before proceeding to step four.

**FOURTH:**

Rub in either sesame oil or coconut oil all over face, neck, chest and hands. Be sure to get your lips and under your eyes, too.

**Once a week:**

Do a PORE MINIMIZER treatment before the THIRD step.

## LIST OF INGREDIENTS and SUPPLIES

- Organic, Cold-Pressed, Raw, Extra Virgin Coconut Oil
- Organic, Cold-Pressed, Raw, Ayurveda Sesame Oil
- Lemon
- Organic, Local, Raw Honey[50]
- Organic White Rice
- Buf-Puf Exfoliating Facial Cleansing Sponges
- Spearmint Essential Oil
- Eucalyptus Essential Oil
- Epsom Salt
- Baking Soda
- Body Brush

---

50    Proverbs 16:24 "Pleasant words are a honeycomb, sweet to the soul and healing to the bones."

# *RECIPES*

> **SIDE BAR:** This FACIAL TONER was introduced to me by my sister-outlaw, Claire. If I remember correctly, she said that it's an old Chinese concoction used for centuries. It cools, cleanses, tightens, and tones the face and neck. It works! You can literally feel your face tighten as the starchy liquid dries. It's amazing and very refreshing after a workout or on a hot day. This is my version of the recipe.[51]

## FACIAL TONER

- 1 ½ cups Organic medium or short grain WHITE rice
- 5 cups boiling hot water

Put rice in a bowl and pour hot water over it. Stir the rice and let it soak at least 2 hours (overnight is ok). Strain off the soaking-water into small containers, or an ice cube tray, and place in the freezer. Thaw out a cube or 2 as needed, in the refrigerator. The toner will last up to 1 week in the refrigerator.

*\* Cook the soaked rice and eat immediately or freeze for later use.*

\*<u>Flash Freezing Rice:</u>

Let the cooked rice cool. Line a baking sheet with foil and then parchment paper. Spread out the cooked (cooled) rice in a

---

51 Each morning when I open my eyes I say to myself: I, not events, have the power to make me happy or unhappy today. I can choose which it shall be. Yesterday is dead, tomorrow hasn't arrived yet. I have just one day, today, and I'm going to be happy in it. – Groucho Marx

thin layer on the parchment paper and place it in the freezer for approximately 45 minutes. Transfer the rice to a freezer bag and store in the freezer. Now you have "instant" frozen rice – just microwave, covered, on high for 5 minutes. Remove from the microwave and let steam for 2 minutes before removing the cover, and EAT!

## PORE MINIMIZER

Put a few drops of organic raw honey on the cut end of a lemon wedge. Rub over the affected areas of your face. Leave it on your face for 5 minutes. Rinse with cold water. Do this once a week.

*This treatment moisturizes, has anti-bacterial and anti-inflammatory properties, and helps fade dark spots /sun spots.*

## BATH SOAK

- Epsom Salt
- 3-5 drops Eucalyptus Essential Oil (sinus and allergy relief)
- 3-5 drops Spearmint Essential Oil (sinus and allergy relief)
- Baking Soda

*Essential oils are optional. Use any combinations you like.*

For a standard sized bath tub:

Fill the tub with water that's as hot as you can stand it, and fill it to a level that allows most of your body to be submerged. Add 1-3 cups of Epsom Salt to the tub. (For a large jacuzzi tub, use 3-5 cups.)

Add ¼-1 cup baking soda. (I usually use about ¼ cup). Add Essential Oils if you desire.

Soak for 20-30 minutes. If you have never done an Epsom salt bath before, start with 10 minutes and work your way up to 30 minutes. **If you are sick**, only soak for 10-15 minutes. You may feel worse afterwards if you are sick or in need of a major detox. This is normal.

I suggest doing these baths right before bed. Take 2-3 bath soaks per week.

*Epsom salt is good for: relaxation, muscle soreness, reduces inflammation, helps heal bruises, sleep aid, detoxifies, aids in digestion (bowels), softens and heals dry skin, reduces stress, helps heal sunburns, relieves itchy skin and bug bites/stings, increases magnesium and sulfate blood levels. Epsom salt also has many household cleaning and gardening uses, too!*

## DRY BRUSHING

**Before soaking: DRY BRUSH** *(I recommend a medium bristle brush. Think Goldie-Locks: not too soft. Not too hard. Just right.)* Brush all parts of your body towards your heart. Do not wet the brush or your skin before brushing.

*Dry brushing stimulates the lymphatic system, helps to regulate hormones, exfoliates the skin, increases circula-*

*tion, opens pores, and promotes the detoxification process through the skin.*

## LIP GLOSS[52]

- 1 Tbl. Organic Coconut Oil, melted
- 2-3 drops flavored extract (vanilla, peppermint, root beer, orange, cinnamon)

Put your favorite flavored extract in a lip balm tube or jar and fill the rest of the way up with melted coconut oil. Place it in the refrigerator to set.

*Coconut oil is liquid at temperatures 70° or higher and solid at temperatures under 70°.*

## EYE MASK – DEPUFFER

Place used green tea bags in a Ziploc bag and keep them in the freezer. Place a tea bag over each (closed) eye for 5-10 minutes to reduce puffiness and dark under-eye circles.

## MORE!

Hand sanitizers can be too harsh for those with sensitive skin. Use coconut oil instead of hand sanitizers and lotion. Coconut oil is the best moisturizer with natural sunscreen and antibacterial properties. It heals cuts and scrapes, is an anti-fungal, and great for your nails. It's a great alternative for those who are allergic to sunscreen and fragrances.

---

52    Proverbs 25:11 "A word aptly spoken is like apples of gold in settings of silver."

While I use coconut oil to remove my eye make-up, I alternate between coconut and sesame oils as my facial moisturizer. Sesame oil has the same moisturizing and healing properties as coconut oil.

> **TIP:** *If you have OILY or NORMAL SKIN, or you LIVE in a HUMID CLIMATE, I recommend using COCONUT OIL as your face and neck moisturizer. I know this sounds strange, but it will actually help heal acne due to its antibacterial properties. (The best thing I have ever found for topical "zit cream" is Close-Up Toothpaste. Put a dab on each zit before bed. Plus, it's red! Ha ha.)*
>
> *If you have DRY SKIN, you are in MENOPAUSE or POST-MENOPAUSAL, or you live in a very DRY CLIMATE, I recommend using SESAME OIL as your face and neck moisturizer. It's a little bit heavier than coconut oil. So, you can get the moisturizing benefits with less. If you find that it "sits" on your face, then either use less sesame oil or switch to coconut oil. With a little trial and error, you will find what works best for you.*

I also use **SOAP** without any fragrances. I prefer them be made with food ingredients such as goat's milk, oatmeal, honey, vanilla, coconut oil, ground nuts and fruit pits/seeds which act as exfoliators.

Let's talk **EYELASHES!** My long, thick eyelashes began to thin and fall out due to thyroid issues and menopause. For ten years I have successfully used a non-prescription brand lash enhancer and grower. My eyelashes grow so long, I have to trim them!

I have found that **MAKEUP** made with coconut oil or without fragrance works best for me. Again, I'm happy to share all the brands I currently use if you contact me through my website at www.getfitwithkimtoday.com.

You can have all the magic creams and treatments in the world, but how you treat your body on the inside (nutrition, sleep, stress management, spiritual health) shows up on the outside.

*Real beauty comes from within.*

I encourage you to take a few moments to read Proverbs 31:10-31 to learn how to become a truly beautiful woman all the days of your life.

*"Your beauty should not come from outward adornment, such as braided hair and the wearing of gold jewelry and fine clothes. Instead, it should be that of your inner self, the unfading beauty of a gentle and quiet spirit, which is of great worth in God's sight."*

*1 Peter 3:3-4*

# FAITH

When did we become tainted and associate good health with reward and punishment? Food is not a reward, and exercise is not punishment. Or at least they are not intended to be those things. Contrary to what some people think or say and what the media implies....

**YOUR SIZE DOES NOT EQUAL YOUR WORTH,**
and
**HOW HEALTHY OR UNHEALTHY YOU ARE DOES NOT DETERMINE YOUR LEVEL OF LAZINESS OR WILLPOWER.**

Unfortunately, society likes to put labels on everything, including our health and worth.

I have been skinny. I have been fat. I have been an athlete. I have been completely out-of-shape. I have been healthy, and I have been sick. Such is life. I have tried almost every weight loss strategy, pill, diet, and "magic fix" out there. I have made it my mission to educate myself in nutrition and fitness, not only to help others, but to also "fix" myself. I have dabbled in eating disorders, body building, ultra-endurance sports (sometimes that included eating as a sport by default. Ha!), and giving up. Yes! At one point, I gave up trying to get back to my healthy weight and fitness level. I have felt body shamed: too skinny as a child; too fat as a twirler; too healthy as an adult. For much of my adult life I've viewed myself and my body as the world does – through guilt, shame, and vanity. And you know what I have learned?

**It doesn't now, never has, and never will work to motivate yourself to get healthy if the motivation is coming from a worldly viewpoint.**

If your motivation for weight loss or fitness is solely based on vanity, acceptance[53], winning, respect, or worth; **YOU WILL EVENTUALLY FAIL**. We get physically and mentally exhausted, and those are not good enough reasons to keep us motivated.

**The one and only way that I've clawed my way back to health** is by giving myself and my body to God. Specifically, I changed my perspective about myself and my body from a worldly view to a Godly one. [54]

# THE FOUNDATION OF AN ETERNAL "WHY"

➢ Your body is a *gift* to you *from* God! Your body was made *by* God to be used *for* Him, not for your selfish gain.

➢ God has entrusted you with this temple that is your body to take care of and use to serve Him and others for His glory, not your own.

➢ God sent His one and only Son, Jesus Christ, to die for YOU.

*"Do you not know that your body is a temple of the Holy Spirit, who is in you, whom you have received from God? You are not your own; you were bought at a price. Therefore, honor God with your body." 1 Corinthians 6:19*

We are to be good stewards of our time, our money, the planet, our resources, our kids, and our health is no different. We have

---

53    Galatians 1:10 "Am I now trying to win the approval of men, or of God? Or am I trying to please men? If I were still trying to please men, I would not be a servant of Christ."

54    Romans 12:2 "Do not conform any longer to the pattern of this world, but be transformed by the renewing of your mind. Then you will be able to test and approve what God's will is – His good, pleasing and perfect will."

an obligation and responsibility as believers in Christ to care for our bodies, because it houses the Holy Spirit.

God commands us to care for our bodies, and by doing so we are, in fact, worshipping Him. *"Therefore, I urge you, brothers, in view of God's mercy, to offer your bodies as living sacrifices, holy and pleasing to God – this is your spiritual act of worship."* *Romans 12:1*

As Christians, it's a privilege and an honor to get the opportunity to make a difference in the world and for others around us. How can we do that if we don't take our own health seriously? How can we expect to work, play, study, serve, fellowship, and live life according to God's will for us if we are exhausted, out-of-shape, sick, or just don't feel our best? How can we expect others to treat us with love and respect if we are not caring for ourselves in the most basic ways by taking care of our mind, body, and spirit? Meaning, we don't smoke or drink to excess, rest, exercise, eat nutritiously, manage our stress, study God's word, etc., to name a few? I think the Apostle Paul said it best in *Romans 8:1-13*.

> *"Therefore, there is now no condemnation for those who are in Christ Jesus, because through Christ Jesus the law of the Spirit who gives life has set you free from the law of sin and death. For what the law was powerless to do because it was weakened by the flesh, God did by sending his own Son in the likeness of sinful flesh to be a sin offering. And so he condemned sin in the flesh, in order that the righteous requirement of the law might be fully met in us, who do not live according to the flesh but according to the Spirit.*

*Those who live according to the flesh have their minds set on what the flesh desires; but those who live in accordance with the Spirit have their minds set on what the Spirit desires. The mind governed by the flesh is death, but the mind governed by the Spirit is life and peace. The mind governed by the flesh is hostile to God; it does not submit to God's law, nor can it do so. Those who are in the realm of the flesh cannot please God.*

*You, however, are not in the realm of the flesh but are in the realm of the Spirit, if indeed the Spirit of God lives in you. And if anyone does not have the Spirit of Christ, they do not belong to Christ. But if Christ is in you, then even though your body is subject to death because of sin, the Spirit gives life because of righteousness. And if the Spirit of him who raised Jesus from the dead is living in you, he who raised Christ from the dead will also give life to your mortal bodies because of his Spirit who lives in you. Therefore, brothers and sisters, we have an obligation—but it is not to the flesh, to live according to it. For if you live according to the flesh, you will die; but if by the Spirit you put to death the misdeeds of the body, you will live."*

## FOOD IS POWERFUL.

To not recognize this is dangerous. Let me explain....

Food has the ability to:

- bring people together – Holiday meals, celebrations, meetings, important discussions, compromises, world leaders

- tear people apart – world hunger, vegans vs. meat eaters, religious beliefs and practices, and dare I say, "DIETS"
- cause wars – the Boston Tea Party, The Salt War, The Serbian Pork War
- spark treaties – resolutions of said wars
- comfort – funerals, Mom's cooking, friends love
- heal you – fruits, veggies
- kill you – fast food, over-consumption

## FOOD IS AN IMPORTANT PART OF OUR SPIRITUAL CULTURE

To ignore the spiritual aspect and connection to nutrition, fitness, and health is to also ignore, remove, and degrade the importance of food and its connections to *everything*. We put far too little importance on our health and its relationship to our faith and salvation.

**When we ignore our health, we disrespect the gift and purpose of our body.**

In studying the Bible, we recognize how God uses food throughout – its taste, our body's daily need for it, it's connections to memory and learning, etc. – to teach us, warn us, guide us, fill us, satisfy us, connect us. Food is used to demonstrate obedience and rebellion. We are told to pray over our food, fast, reap and sow, sacrifice, share and feed those less fortunate.

**Here are just a few examples of how food is used to:**

- Tempt us | APPLE (Genesis 3)
- Test our faith and dependence on God | MANNA (Exodus 16)
- Challenge us | DANIEL (Daniel 1)
- Grow us (faith) | MUSTARD SEED, YEAST (Matthew 13)
- Provide for us | FEEDING THE 5000 (Luke 9)
- SAVE US (CHRIST'S BODY) | BREAD AND WINE (Luke 22), LIVING WATER (John 7)

God compares life and its challenges to a "race" (1 Corinthians 9:24) and other physical feats (Isaiah 40:31). Jesus Christ is referred to as "The Bread of Life." If God equated food to our Savior, Jesus, shouldn't we be more diligent in how *we* relate to and use food?

We cannot live without it, but for some food can be a double-edged sword. We abuse food just as we abuse other things. God intends for us to enjoy food and use it to help us celebrate, comfort others, unite people, etc. However, He does not intend for us to use food to *replace* Him. Nor does God intend for us to abuse food.

*1 Corinthians 6:13a "...Food for the stomach and the stomach for food, but God will destroy them both."*

FOOD IS FUNDAMENTALLY THE ONE THING THAT
CONNECTS EVERY HUMAN ON THE PLANET.

Why does God use food, exercise, illness, and health to teach us life lessons? Because everyone – big, small, young, old, sick, healthy, of all backgrounds, cultures, and colors – eats, feels hunger, needs food and exercise, gets sick, etc. Not everyone relates to sports, or books, or music. While great ways to witness to others, they only reach a small demographic.

On the other hand, food crosses borders, race, gender, age, socio-economic backgrounds, oceans, education.

WE CAN ALL RELATE TO FOOD NO MATTER OUR
LOCATION OR BELIEFS.
It's UNIVERSAL.

God designed it that way for a reason. The gift of salvation is available to *all* who are willing to receive it.[55] How did His disciples spread the news of this amazing gift and need for Jesus Christ? By sharing a meal with others! Jesus even did this with his closest friends – the Last Supper - before His crucifixion where He introduced bread (the body of Christ) and wine (the blood of Christ). Food was significant enough for God to use it to represent His one and only Son. The Son of man and of God! *"The Bread of Life." (John 6:35)*

Knowing this, how can we continue to abuse food and exercise? How can we continue to neglect our health? How can we continue to abuse our bodies? **Once we have this knowledge, know our purpose, and receive Jesus as our Savior, we should feel an undeniable responsibility to care for our bodies in the way God intended.** Not for our own sake and vanity, but for the work and purpose God planned for us. Now, I'm not saying this easy. We are imperfect and live in an imperfect world. Temptation is *real*. But knowing this and changing our

---

55   John 3:16 "For God so loved the world that He gave His only begotten Son, that whosoever believes in Him shall not perish but have eternal life."

perspective can give us the power to resist it. Not by our own power, but *with* God's power.

Food is an issue for EVERYONE: either you personally, or someone you know, suffers with some form of food-related issue. As Christians, we have an amazing opportunity to witness simply by taking care of our bodies. But this is hard.

## MY STORY:

For many years, the need to be viewed as a "fit, have-it-all-together expert" in my field of fitness and nutrition, is what drove me – drove me to study and get education and certifications. Drove me to exercise and diet obsessively. Drove me to compete in triathlons and become a triathlon coach. And I did have a high level of success. I had the most successful aerobics classes and programs in my city for many years. I helped hundreds of people get in shape through my aerobics classes, personal training, triathlon and coaching programs for running, diet and nutrition.

I thought I would lose my influence to help others get healthy and lose weight if I was not the "perfect" living physical proof of a healthy lifestyle. Being a fitness professional, I put tremendous pressure on myself to have the perfect outward appearance. As a result, I was miserable, despite my success as a fitness professional and athlete. I found myself exhausted, injured, discouraged, and frustrated. And you know what? My projection of "perfection" isolated me and left me with little influence.

Because others viewed me as someone who could not

possibly understand their struggles with weight loss, my biggest fear came true. I couldn't help anyone because I became unapproachable.

Little did they know my dirty little secret:

I struggled *constantly* with my weight, self-confidence, laziness, and my health – physically, mentally, and spiritually.

Finally, I reached the point that I gave up trying to be the "epitome of health." I was just plain exhausted – physically and mentally. I distinctly remember asking myself this question, **"If this is as good as I'm going to be – weight, fitness, business – can I live and be happy with that?"** My sad little answer was *"no."*

For the next 16 months, I prayed a simple but very significant prayer. I'm not sure where it came from. Wait, I take that back. I do know where it came from. It came from the Holy Spirit. Anyway, several times a day I prayed:

*"God, help me see myself the way You see me."*

Later, He added to that prayer,

*"And God, help me see others the way You see them."*

And later still, He added,

*"And God, help me see You for who You truly are."*

The healing, wisdom, discernment, and compassion and love for others, myself, and God brought by those simple prayers can't be fully expressed. Praying sincerely this way completely changed my life. God came through, as always, and answered slowly but surely every single one of those three prayers.

About 16 months later, I asked myself the question again. ***"If this is as good as I'm going to be – weight, fitness, business – can I live and be happy with that?"***

My joyous answer was *"yes!"* Not because I gave up on my health—but because I knew God had given me understanding. He led me to realize He could use me more to help others while *in* my struggle than in any other vision I had for myself. The fact was I wanted desperately to be used by God. Whatever that meant for me personally, I was (and am still) willing to sacrifice whatever He desires to follow His path.

Flash forward another year. I still struggled with being 30-40 lbs. overweight. Still struggled to find the perfect cocktail of supplements and medications that (with my doctor's guidance) would keep me healthy. Surprisingly, I found myself living with a peace and confidence that I have *never* experienced before. One with amazing depth and comfort surpassing my understanding. That peace and confidence allowed me to realize my *ETERNAL "WHY"* and to set goals reflecting *that* "WHY."

Until my thinking and perspective changed, I was unable to quit fighting myself. I was unable to see my unique worth – worth in Christ. When I quit fighting, my heart opened, and God showed me the way. I know the same is true for you: until you're thinking and perspective changes, you will not be able to find your *Eternal "WHY."*

## THE PLANNING PHASE - GOAL SETTING:

So much has been written about how to set goals and achieve them. They all seem to have the same formula to success wrapped up in a slightly different package. I won't try to reinvent the wheel. These strategies work because they all have a common thread:

YOU MUST SET GOALS

and

YOU MUST HAVE A PLAN TO REACH THOSE GOALS

This lesson in life is laid out for us in Proverbs 4:25-27

➤ *"Let your eyes look straight ahead, fix your gaze directly before you."*

TRANSLATION: Set goals for yourself.

➤ *"Make level paths for your feet and take only ways that are firm."*

TRANSLATION: Have a plan and prepare for success.

➤ *"Do not swerve to the right or the left; keep your foot from evil."*

TRANSLATION: Be steadfast and stand firm. Remove and avoid temptations and distractions.

> **SIDE BAR:** *These scriptural references are cited with health and wellness in mind. By no means do any of the scriptures I reference throughout this book ONLY relate to health, food, and goals. All the suggestions, points, and references from these scriptures are intended by God to be used in every area of our lives.*

One of my favorite quotes is by Roger Halston:

*"When you work at the little things, big things happen."*

This is goal setting summed up in a nut shell. No matter what overwhelming goal you have – losing 100 lbs., competing in an Ironman Triathlon, walking down the hall after surgery, changing careers, going back to school, saving for retirement—breaking it down into small, manageable tasks is the only way to make it happen. Here are some strategies to help get you going on a life-changing journey to your dreams:

## LEARN HOW TO SET GOALS

**Goals must be:**

- **SPECIFIC:** Know *exactly* what you are working towards. If you want to lose weight, your goal should state, "I want to lose blank lbs. by such-and-such date."

- **ATTAINABLE:** Be able to complete and reach your goal in a realistic timeframe. For example: no one can lose 100 lbs. in a month. Set yourself up for success, not failure.

- **REALISTIC:** Make your goal within your reach. You cannot race in a triathlon if you cannot afford a bicycle.

- **TRACKABLE:** Track and review your progress. We all

get discouraged if we cannot see how far we've come. It's easier to keep going if you can see progress along the way. JOURNALING is the best way to do this successfully.

- **SHORT TERM:** We all need "benchmark" goals (or "mile markers" as I like to call them). The little successes along the way to our ultimate long-term goal provide motivation to keep going. For example: running three miles in two months is moving in the right direction toward the long-term goal of running a marathon.

- **LONG TERM:** These goals are in the future – a year or more away.

- **PLANNED:** PLAN, PLAN, PLAN!

For some of us, this is the fun part. For others, it's torture, but for *everyone,* it's necessary. Without a plan, you will not succeed in any area you want to change. [56]Habits are ingrained in us - sometimes for years - which is why they are hard to break.[57] Sometimes, they may even seem impossible to break. Having a structure and a plan set in place helps ensure good options available to you.

For example, you will be less likely to hit the drive-thru window if you're starving, because you have a "snack pack" filled with healthy foods in your car. Or you have a big pot of veggie soup and cooked chicken already waiting for you in your fridge. If you set a workout time with a friend or trainer, you are more likely to keep it. If you decide to brush your teeth after every meal, but don't have a toothbrush in your

---

56  "By failing to prepare, you are preparing to fail." Benjamin Franklin

57  "Habit is habit and not to be flung out of the window by any man, but coaxed downstairs a step at a time." Mark Twain

desk/car/purse— then you aren't likely to make that a new habit. Make it happen by planning ahead.

Figure out what a realistic schedule and plan is for you. Find someone to join you or hire someone to help you reach those goals by holding you accountable. And finally, get to work!

- **YOUR GOALS MUST REFLECT YOUR "WHY."**

## HAVE AN ETERNAL "WHY" THAT LEADS TO EVERLASTING CHANGE

Your "WHY" matters not only to your own success in reaching and keeping your goals but also to God and His purpose for your life.

### *This is the biggest take-a-way from the entire book!*

How many times have you seen someone lose a lot of weight for a big event, only to quickly gain it back after that event was over? The problem wasn't their "WHY" – lose weight for my daughter's wedding, for example. There was obviously motivation in that "WHY," because the goal was reached. The problem lies in that it wasn't an *eternal* "WHY." There was no motivation to continue *after* the event passed. To make lifelong *changes* in any area, our main "WHY" must be bigger than our own "selfish gain."

### To have EVERLASTING CHANGE, you must have an *Eternal "WHY."*

We've seen the ads, posts, blogs, and testimonies of those who have quit something, like smoking, for example. Typically, they do it for health reasons. Most say something like, "Everything changed when I had a child. I had a reason to quit." The key here is that before then, they never had a good enough "selfish" reason to quit *forever*. (Actually, if you don't quit "forever," you never really, quit. You technically just took a break.) If selfish gain – looking good, impressing someone, feeling better, winning, etc. - was a good enough reason, then we could all be "fixed" and never need any help with anything.

## If you have a SUPERFICIAL "WHY," your results will be temporary.

**The FIRST STEP** in everlasting change and lifelong results is figuring out the underlying cause of your distress, which is leading you to cope in an unhealthy way. For instance, if you are morbidly obese, then find the root of *why you are overeating*. Trust me; there is a reason, other than hunger, that you are overeating. There is a reason why you are smoking, drinking, or doing drugs, other than being "social."

There is a reason why you do the things you do – good and bad, healthy and unhealthy – and those reasons become apparent in the way you work, play, relax, worship, relate to others, and look. Whether you realize it or not, **your outside appearance reflects the physical, mental, and spiritual health of your insides.** They are all interrelated. Realizing the significance of this and how it translates into why you do *everything* is eye – and heart – opening. In my experience, when one of these three – Fitness, Food, or Faith - are off track, the others soon follow. It's a clear indication that I'm relying on myself, others, food, exercise, or anything other than God, for my strength and comfort.

## MY STORY:

For many years, I was very competitive in triathlons. While I was not a good swimmer, cyclist, or runner, the law of averages was in my favor. I won my fair share of 1st, 2nd, and 3rd place trophies in my age group. I even won first place in the "Overall Female" category at a race. I completed two 70.3 Ironman Triathlons as well as countless Sprint and Olympic distance triathlons. To those on the outside looking in, my racing, career, and life looked picturesque.

*I have never been so mentally and physically exhausted and miserable in my entire life.*

There were things going on in my personal life that I didn't know how to deal with – things I, quite frankly, didn't want to deal with. My solution was to be so physically exhausted from triathlon training 20+ hours a week on top of my job and life responsibilities, that I didn't have to think about, or deal with any issue or problem.

I thought I was being a strong, independent, leader by trying to do everything myself. I thought if I worked hard enough, tried hard enough, wanted it bad enough, I would eventually get "it." Whatever "it" was.

Without realizing it, I was living by my own rules and relying on my own strength and abilities to "get through" things instead of asking God to help, show, and provide a way for me. I was living through works instead of grace and love – which is God's way. That, my friends, was why I was so exhausted and losing everything. Fortunately, it drove me to the brink of losing it all. Yes, I wrote *"FORTUNATELY."*

God used it all to bring me to my knees, literally, and face everything I had been avoiding. He loved me enough to not let me continue down that path and completely took away my physical ability to do *everything* by myself; walk, shop, housework, cook, bathe, and even wash my hair.

**SIDE BAR:** I was born with severe flat feet and a slight deformity in my left foot which caused me great pain and many injuries throughout my life. I never let it really inhibit me much, but my foot finally did "fail." I couldn't stand on that leg. I was in constant pain, and I could no longer come up on my toes with that foot. (On my own, I had strengthened my body to support the dysfunctional foot, researched, and made inquiries to several profes-sionals about what to do with my foot. To no avail.) Only after I couldn't walk for several days after racing my last 70.3 Ironman Triathlon, was I able to find a foot specialist familiar with my specific problem. My Doc finally said it was time for the surgery after a year of physical therapy, six months of traction therapy to stretch my Achilles tendon, and a specially made and designed traction brace made by a prosthetic company. (I traveled back and forth to Austin every two weeks for more than two years.) He had done all the individual components to the surgery before, just not on one foot at the same time. I was the "Surgical Procedure to Watch." It took five hours, but he built me a new foot! The recovery was hard and LONG. I was not able to put *any* weight on that foot for three months. This meant I was *completely dependent on* *everyone else for everything.* I had to let all my pride[58] and independence go. It forced me to not only *ask* for help but *accept* help from others. I learned it was just as much a blessing for them to be able to help as it was for me receiving the help. It completely changed my life, allowing God to "work" on me because I was finally *still.*[59]

One thing I did during my recovery ("still") time was read a chapter in Psalms every day. There are 150 chapters, taking me 150 days to read. It not only lifted my spirits but also changed my prayer life and perspective. If you are new to reading the Bible and don't know where to begin, I recommend starting with Psalms.

God took away the "healthy" thing – triathlon – I was using to replace Him. In doing so, He led me back to Him and healed me physically, mentally, emotionally, relationally, and spiritually. It has been a process; a long, difficult road paved with tears. A growing change in every way for the past six years, because as dynamic as the foot surgery was, it was not the end of my health struggle.

Looking back, the verses in 2 Corinthians 4:16-17 have come to life in a real and glorious way for me.

> *"Therefore, we do not lose heart. Though outwardly we are wasting away, yet inwardly we are being renewed day by day. For our light and momentary troubles are achieving for us an eternal glory that far outweighs them all."*

---

58 Daniel 4:37 says "He is able to humble those who walk in pride."

59 Psalm 46: 10 "Be still and know that I am God;"

I know I am not finished yet, but the ride is no longer scary due to verse 18....

> *"So, we fix our eyes not on what is seen, but on what is unseen. For what is seen is temporary, but what is unseen is eternal."*

Once you understand *why* you do something, then you can go to **STEP 2:**

*SURRENDER IT TO GOD.*

He alone can heal your pain, comfort you, motivate you, give you purpose, and save you. [60] *Once you know your purpose, you have the knowledge to find your Eternal "WHY," and nothing and no one can stop you.* You will have everlasting results, because your "WHY" also becomes your testimony – glorifying Christ and not yourself – aligning your purpose with your "WHY." This is the *healthy* reason you are doing what you do to fulfill your true purpose.

**THE THIRD STEP** is to *Get Out of Your Own Way*. You, first and foremost, need a plan to reach your goals. This is where I typically get stuck. I plan and plan and plan, but when it comes time to take *action*, I become paralyzed. I allow fear and negativity to seep into my thoughts.

> "Can I really do this?"
> "What if I fail?"
> "What will everyone think if I'm not able to do it?"

---

60   "The two most important days of your life are the day you were born, and the day you find out why." – Mark Twain

Then I procrastinate, saying to myself...

"Maybe I'm not quite ready."
"I need more _____ before I start."
"I'll do this without telling anyone I'm doing it, just *in case*
I fail. I don't really need anyone to help me or hold me
accountable."

And my famous last words....

"I got this. I can do this on my own."
**WRONG!**

God wants your health – *your life* – to reflect Him. He will NEVER have your high school reunion, daughter's wedding, or any other "self-serving" desire be *THE essential "WHY"* that gets you long-term results. *It must be bigger than yourself.* When your "WHY" aligns with His will, your desires will align with His desires for you.

Psalm 37:4 says, *"Take delight in the Lord, and He will give you the desires of your heart."* When fear and doubt creep into your thoughts, remember 2 Timothy 1:7 *"God did not give us a spirit of fear, but a spirit of power, of love, and of self-discipline."*

# HOW TO START AND WHERE TO BEGIN

## "DAY 1"

Day 1 has typically been a toe stumper for me in the past. I could never quite seem to get past "Day 1." I'd start whatever plan I decided was right for me at the time, do great until about day four, and "mess up." My perfectionist attitude didn't allow for the occasional toe stump, trip, or fall. So, "DAY 1" eventually rolled around again and again.

Finally, my insightful (sometimes annoyingly so) husband said, "STOP STARTING OVER! THERE IS NO MORE DAY 1!" That resonated with me. I discovered that many others also kept finding themselves at "DAY 1" over and over and over. What a defeating lifestyle! This got me thinking... if the *meaning* of "DAY 1" changed, then none of us would ever have to revisit "DAY 1" again!

### WHAT IS the *NEW* "DAY 1?"

DAY 1 is the day you write down your *eternal WHY*, set *goals*, and make your *plan* to help you reach those goals. [61]

THAT'S IT! You do *nothing* else on "DAY 1." It is reserved for getting *prepared* to START.

---

61   Proverbs 16:3 "Commit to the Lord whatever you do, and He will establish your plans."

## DAY 2 is the day you TAKE ACTION!

All the learning, reading, and planning is meaningless until you take the first step into ACTION.[62] You could have the magic weight loss pill in your hand, but if you never swallow it, then it won't work. It takes WORK to change and become successful. It takes sweat, tears (sometimes lots of tears), perseverance, discipline, endurance, falling down, and getting back up to make change happen.

Your health is a LABOR of LOVE.

A love for the *gift* God has blessed you with.

**FOOD FOR THOUGHT:**

Let's say everyone is given one vehicle for their entire life. Some people get a van, some get a sports car, some get a jacked up pick-up truck, and others get a Mini Cooper. Everyone gets a unique vehicle all their own to use as they like for their entire life. There's no trading, and no two are alike.

Would you put bad gas in your vehicle? Would you put bald tires on your vehicle? Would you leave it sitting in the garage for decades and then take it out on an icy race track at high speeds? Would you expect it to be safe and run well if you neglected it in any way? Of course not!

Now, let's say...

Your body is that vehicle.

*You get one life to live and one body to carry you through that life.*

---

62  "Just Do It!" ~ Nike

- What do you want to accomplish with this one life?
- Are you caring for your body in a way that is going to allow that life to happen?
- Are you living up to your full potential?
- Is your health holding you back?
- How do you think God feels about the way you treat your body? Not just physically, but also mentally in how you *think* about your body?

When you begin to view your body as an amazing gift God specifically designed *just for you*, then amazing transformations happen. God put a lot of thought and effort to make you *special* and *unique*. Honor Him and His gift by taking *special* care of it.

*The goal should not be to achieve perfection,*
*but to let others see how you live with and work through your*
*imperfections.*

Periodically, we should ask ourselves the questions above to keep us on the right track. It's easy to recognize how we may neglect our health, but these questions also help those who tend to take something healthy and abuse it, causing an unhealthy result.

## YOU MUST BELIEVE IN ORDER TO RECEIVE

There is a big difference between *knowing* and *believing*.

You can *know* about a lot of things. For example: You can *know* weight loss is possible. You can *know* being healthy is possible. You can *know* running a marathon is possible. You can *know* beating cancer is possible. You can *know* God loves you and has the best plans for you.

However, until you *BELIEVE* anything imaginable is possible you will never reach your highest goals and expectations - or God's expectations for your life.

Until you *BELIEVE* total health and wellness – spiritual, emotional, physical, and everything that encompasses for you – is possible....

Until you *BELIEVE* all your hopes and dreams will be revealed and come to fruition....

Until you *BELIEVE* not only those things *are* possible, but that God *wants* them for you....

> *you will never fully reach those dreams.*

You may have small, short-lived successes, but they will *always* be followed by setbacks.

> The missing link to long-term success
> and
> lifelong health and wellness is the
> BELIEF
> it's possible
> and
> you can achieve it.

Once you *believe* God and *believe* He wants you to be healthy - physically, emotionally and spiritually - you will find a peace you've never experienced before. Your faith will grow like it has never grown before, because you *believed* and *asked* with confidence – confidence in the Lord.[63] Everything starts with a thought, a dream, a hope, a wish, an idea. It's followed by a desire for knowledge, learning, and planning. Ultimately, that's followed by action[64], perseverance, and faith. Finally...

### YOU BELIEVE and YOU RECEIVE.

Believing change is possible comes in stages, with small successes along the way, as you WORK towards your goals. We need these small successes to increase our faith and motivate us.

*"If you believe, you will receive whatever you ask for in prayer." Matthew 21:22*

## FINDING THE MOTIVATION TO START

Many of you are having a difficult time finding the motivation to get off the couch and start exercising (or whatever your goal is). Somehow, losing the weight, lowering cholesterol, running the marathon in three months, or getting your doctor (or spouse) off your back, just isn't enough to get you going. Maybe you've been inconsistent in your workouts or dieting; having an attitude like the guy in the Nicorette Patch commercial who says, "I've quit smoking for 15 days. Just not in a row." I think we can all relate. Or, do you have a case of "I'll start tomorrow." Well friends, yesterday you said "tomorrow." And guess what?

### *TODAY IS TOMORROW*

---

63    Hebrews10:35 "So do not throw away your confidence; it will be richly rewarded."

64    James 1:22 "Do not merely listen to the word, and so deceive yourselves. Do what it says."

First, be ok with where you are starting, today. Don't compare yourself to anyone else. Everyone has their own road to walk. Take that first step. Right now! You will never regret it. You will only regret the time lost before you took that very first step towards health – i.e. freedom.

I have never heard anyone say, "Man, I wish I had waited longer to start _____." One of my favorite authors, Lysa Terkherst, wrote "Whether you succeed or fail is determined by the very next choice you make." Will your next choice be one leading you down the path toward your goals or away from them?

## FINDING THE MOTIVATION TO KEEP GOING[65]

*Motivation is what gets you started. Habit is what keeps you going. ~ Jim Ryun*

Without a destination, the road to success will be at best bumpy, and at worst a dead end. Maybe you've lost sight of your goal. Maybe you reached your first goal and need to set another one. Maybe your goal has changed or was never specific or realistic. Whatever the case may be, take time to review, reflect, and/or readjust a goal to work towards.

We think of January as the only time to set goals – New Year's Resolutions. However, ANY TIME is the perfect time to start setting goals. After six months, revisit and reevaluate.

Sometimes a change in priorities or circumstances that are out of you control, can cause you to not be able to achieve a goal or need to postpone it. Eliminating a goal altogether may be

---

65   Hebrews 10:36 "You need to persevere so that when you have done the will of God, you will receive what he has promised."

necessary. Whatever the case, reevaluating and adjusting your goals at the six-month mark will help you refocus and give you a good sense of how far you've come. It can kick you into high gear if needed. It's easy to get discouraged if you can't see the progress you've made, but if you are tracking your goals through *journaling*, it's easier to stay motivated and make necessary adjustments so you can reach them.

**The key is JOURNALING.** There is no greater accountability tool than writing down a goal you want to achieve. Literally seeing your goals brings them to life, making them either seem possible or unimportant. They can also be written on your bathroom mirror so they're visible every day! Listing goals makes prioritizing them easier. Then develop a plan to accomplish the most important ones, first.

Goal setting and tracking is not the only use for journaling.

## MY STORY:

Not only did journaling help diagnose me but also helped *save* me.

Initially, I began journaling consistently after I had reconstructive foot surgery. I journaled my physical therapy, progress, and nutrition. It started out innocent enough. But tracking my progress led to revealing more about health issues that had been unrecognized by doctors for years. As discussed in earlier chapters, these issues quickly reared their ugly heads.

Journaling allowed me to reflect on past entries and remember that despite my eating a strict and nutritionally-sound diet, my hormones and thyroid still "dumped" (the doctor's term) and quit working properly.

Reflecting helped me stay the course with my treatment and medication plan. Coming to grips with the fact that I *needed* to take medications to LIVE was an extremely difficult process. For the first two years, I was convinced I could eventually get off all medications and maintain my health through proper nutrition. I came to realize that was not true, nor possible. Like so many others, I need medication to function properly and live a healthy, long life. And that's ok.

However, I can *support* the necessary medications with proper nutrition and exercise. Journaling helps keep everything on track and quickly reveal any issues that may need to be addressed *before* they become big health issues.

**SIDE BAR:** In addition to Journaling, I had a small group of five people who I trusted to keep me on track spiritually and emotionally. They helped me stay the course when my treatment plan seemed like it would never fall into place. They were Christians who shared my beliefs and values; who knew me and would still love me despite me; whose input and opinions I respected and trusted; and most importantly who I would listen to! I call them my "Circle of Trust," as Robert De Niro coined in the movie, "Meet the Parents." Ladies (and Gentlemen), do not try to go through hormonal issues, menopause, or any health issue, ALONE!

I know you think people will judge you, think you've gone

nuts, or that you will lose all your friends. As hard as it is to go through a physical malady with a support system, it's impossible to get through it alone. You need support.

I'm not suggesting you plaster all your troubles and thoughts on social media. Be selective in who you invite into your "Circle of Trust." God uses people to help one another in times of need. It's just as therapeutic for others to be needed as it is for you to need their help and guidance. They are also being blessed. You don't want to rob anyone of their blessing. God will bring you through troubles of your own so, in turn, you will be able to help someone else through their tough time. Your testimony becomes someone else's HOPE. That's why it's a CIRCLE.

## HOW TO JOURNAL

There are several phone apps and devices that allow you to record your food, exercise, sleep, and whatever else you want to track for health purposes. Some apps also allow you to type notes, "how you feel," etc. I'm old school, and there's something about hand-writing in a journal that's cathartic for me. Plus, I'm not too keen on having all my info in an app where I might lose the data.

**Here's my system:**

Every year, I buy a different colored spiral notebook. Some years I fill up three notebooks. Other years I may only get half a notebook filled. They are always labeled, and I use a different color each year for quick reference. If I do use an app or tracker, I also record that info into my written journal. Everything is in one place and easily accessible.

There is healing, motivation, and diagnostic benefits to reflection.[66] Sometimes, knowing what is NOT working is more important than figuring out what does work. Patterns arise and become clear. You will be able to quickly see where you got off track and what you were doing when your health was going strong.

Whatever you choose to use as your journal – online, app, tracker, or notebook – there are some key things to track, at least periodically. (Some may or may not apply to you.)

- Sleep
- Weight
- Exercise
  - Type
  - Duration
  - Steps taken
- Food and water/drinks
  - Timing of meals
- Digestive issues
  - How you feel after eating: gas, bloating, upset tummy, headache, etc.
  - Bowel movements – yea or nay
- Medications
  - Timing of medications
  - Side effects

---

66    Psalm 77:11b-12 "...yes, I will remember your miracles of long ago. I will consider all your works and meditate on all your mighty deeds."

- ◦ Helping or not
- Other:
  - ◦ Goals
  - ◦ How you feel/emotions
  - ◦ Gratitude list
  - ◦ Significant events
  - ◦ Struggles
  - ◦ Successes
  - ◦ Menstrual cycle
  - ◦ Blood pressure
  - ◦ Heart rate

## IN ADDITION TO JOURNALING

I highly advise you to begin a *MEDICAL HISTORY FOLDER*. Use this to keep track of all your lab tests, blood pressure readings, health care provider appointments, medications, etc. You'd be surprised how much we rely on memory and how inaccurate it is!

If you happen to be a little Type A+++ like me, you may already have saved your bloodwork from previous years. If not, it's never too late to start.

## MY STORY

Along with my journals, having a comprehensive MEDICAL HISTORY FOLDER of all my bloodwork and tests is what ultimately helped diagnose me. When I did finally find a specialized Endocrinologist who listened, he was able to use my "past" (journals and bloodwork records dating back to my mid-20's) to connect the dots and determine that I had, in fact, gone through menopause in my late 20's. Previous diagnoses stated I was "over-trained" and suffering from extreme low body fat from ultra-endurance training. Those doctors had not taken my symptoms seriously. (To be fair, it's very uncommon for a woman to go through menopause at 26 years of age, but no one ever tested me for hormone issues or thyroid dysfunction, despite my multiple requests, and the fact thyroid dysfunction ran in my family.)

Had I been tested earlier, my diagnosis of Premature Ovarian Failure and Hypothyroidism - along with the treatments thereof - may have not been so extreme, nor taken so long to find the right medications at correct dosages.

Be Your Own Advocate. If something is not working for you; if you feel something is not "right," find a doctor who will listen and do what's necessary to figure out what is going on.

I recommend *every* woman have annual bloodwork starting at age 21, *even if you feel great and are not suffering from any illness.* (Actually, I should write, *"ESPECIALLY if you feel great and are not suffering from any illness."*) If, and when, you do begin having hormone issues, you will be able to have an accurate starting point, instead of a trial and error shot-gun approach to find the correct dosage. It took about four years for my doctor to get the right cocktail of hormones and thyroid medications to find my "happy" place. It did happen, but there were times I literally thought I was going to die. Finding the right doctor as well as the right medications and dosages is key.

## BLOODWORK TO GET TESTED ANNUALLY:

NOTE: You must request to be tested for these.

- Glucose
- Insulin
- TSH
- T3
- T4
- FSH
- LH
- Estradiol
- Progesterone
- Testosterone
- DHEA
- Sodium
- Magnesium
- Potassium
- Zinc
- Cholesterol
- Triglycerides
- Calcium
- Vitamin D3

As your weight fluctuates up or down (hopefully down!), so do your hormones. Adipose tissue (fat) stores and produces hormones, like estrogen. It's a good idea to have your hormone levels checked periodically through blood tests, especially if you are on Hormone Replacement Therapy, thyroid medications, or any other medications related to physical health, like blood pressure, diabetes, or cholesterol. This allows your doctor to make any necessary adjustments to your medications.

I recommend you get your bloodwork rechecked after six months of starting an exercise and nutrition program. If you are losing significant amounts of weight – 25 lbs. or more – and you are on any medication, have your bloodwork redone in 8-12 weeks.

## WHAT TO DO WITH THE RESULTS: Making Your Medical History Folder

1) Once you have done your bloodwork, request a copy of everything (not just the "results" or "readings" from your doctor).

2) Include any other tests/procedures like colonoscopies, irregular pap smears, etc. that may be relative to your future health.

3) Make 1-2 copies.

4) Write how much you weighed and how you "felt" at the time. For example, I know the hormone levels when "I've felt the best I've ever felt!" because I literally wrote that on my lab results copy! In turn, I also know where my levels where when I've felt the worst. This helps you and your doctor know where your "happy place" is and give

a clearer starting point for medications, if the need ever arises.

> **NOTE:** if you are also journaling, you can review those to see if your health issue is linked to exercise, sleep, and/or nutrition. Sometimes, it's a simple fix!

5) Highlight the date the tests were taken for quick reference.

6) Keep copies in one side and originals in the other side of your Medical History Folder.

7) Write your name on the front of your folder and keep it in a safe place, along with your journals.

If you ever fall ill or suffer from hormone-related issues, you will be able to grab your Medical History Folder and quickly make copies for your doctor.

## IT'S NEVER TOO LATE, AND YOU ARE NEVER TOO OLD TO START

But there is a sense of URGENCY. Or at least there should be. How you treat others and yourself (physically, mentally, spiritually) in *this* decade will determine your level of health, happiness, and success in the next decade.

*Did you grasp that statement?*

**You will reap in the NEXT decade of your life what you sow in THIS decade.**

No one knows what the future holds, but you can lay good foundations of health *today* in preparation for the future. The healthy steps you take nutritionally, physically, spiritually, emotionally, etc. *right now,* better your chances of **avoiding or successfully battling** the inevitable health crises that are going to come your way.

No one is immune to disease or injury. There are environmental factors, genetics, and things that, frankly, are out of our control that contribute to disease. However, if you are as healthy as you can possibly be - by controlling the foods you eat, activity during the day, stress levels, etc. – then you will be able to handle, recover from, and possibly avoid the seriousness of some diseases and health problems that arise throughout a lifetime. The healthier you are *prior* to any unfortunate health problem, surgery, or accident, the *quicker* you will recover. The chances of a *full recovery* are *greatly increased,* as well as the likelihood that it will not dramatically affect your life in the future. Do everything you can, now, so when you get hurt or sick, you have a chance of living through it and bouncing back 100%. It's like saving money for a rainy day or planning for retirement. You don't want to wait until disaster strikes, or retirement, before you start.

My question to you is, *"How do you want to live the next decade of your life?"*

I encourage you to read the book of Joshua. Joshua is one of my favorite people in the Bible because he was "middle-aged" when he got his *eternal WHY.* Joshua 14:7 *"I was FORTY YEARS OLD when Moses the servant of the Lord sent me...."* Later in verses 10-11, *"Now then, just as the Lord promised, He has kept me alive.... So here I am today, eighty-five years old!"* [Here's my favorite part!] *"I am still as strong today as the day Moses sent me out; I'm just as vigorous to go out to battle now as I was* then." WHY? Because verse 14b, *"...he [Joshua] followed the Lord, the God of Israel, WHOLEHEARTEDLY."* Now, that's the story I want!

## CREATING THE "NEW" YOU

The Bible says, *"we take off our old selves"* and *"put on our new selves."* We are renewed in Christ. We are quick to accept this in many areas of our life. We are willing to accept this and let go of drug addictions, alcohol addictions, other addictions, our attitudes, perspectives, the way we treat others, etc. Why is it so difficult to think God wants us to claim this promise from Him that we are new and healed regarding our health as well?

Creating new habits is incredibly difficult. It seems it's even more difficult when changing health habits. We start eating nutritiously, and suddenly, we are overwhelmed with "life." Therefore, because it's so new to us, our efforts go out the window, and we revert to our old ways of grabbing fast food. I don't know how many times I have had a client call me and say, "I got really busy, and I was really bad this week. I need to get back on my diet."

*The reason we fall back into old habits is because we don't give enough time for the new habits to get firmly established.*

Make the decision to allow change to happen. Have the courage to stay the course and let the new, *sometimes uncomfortable,* changes become your *new comfortable.*

Don't hold on to your "old" way of doing things or "old" habits. As the saying goes, "Old habits die hard." But they *will die* if you let them. Lay to rest your "old self." Forget about past mistakes.

God has. Forgive yourself for your shortcomings and sins. God has (if you've asked Him). Make the decision today that you are NEW; your attitude is new, your habits are new, your health is new, your life is new.

*Never choose a path or direction you know you cannot maintain for life.* Now, I didn't say never choose a path that was hard. Everything is difficult in the beginning, but to say, "I am never eating chocolate cake again," when that is your favorite birthday cake, is not something you're going to be able to maintain forever. Learn the strategies to help you live a healthy, *balanced* lifestyle. Then you can learn how to incorporate your favorite chocolate birthday cake without derailing your progress and health.

It takes 30 times to change your brain and create new habits. This is not new information. However, what they fail to say is that it takes *at least* 30 times *in a row* to create a new habit.

**STOP!** Did you catch that?

### IT TAKES at least 30 TIMES IN A ROW to create a NEW HABIT!

I like to remind my clients that the extreme soreness and fatigue of starting a new exercise program will generally go away after 30 days. Now they can choose to drag those 30 days out over several months if they only come to work out twice a week. Or, they can exercise daily as I schedule them and get over the initial soreness and fatigue in one month. The choice is theirs. The same is true in other areas as well.

## CHOOSE TO MAKE YOUR DARKEST DAYS YOUR DEFINING MOMENTS

When you're ready to quit and wonder if it really matters if you skip that workout, don't get enough sleep, or have that extra slice of pizza – remember, *IT DOES MATTER*. People are watching you! (Well, hopefully not while you're sleeping! C-R-E-E-P-Y.)

Let your struggle and perseverance be an inspiration and living testimony to others who feel helpless, or that change is impossible. You never know who you are encouraging in their quest to become healthy, just by sticking to your choices and commitment towards good health and continuing in your walk through the obstacles and difficult times.[67] When others may dive head first into a bowl of queso or a gallon of Blue Bell for comfort, you can show them that you choose Jesus to comfort you by *not* indulging in junk food, or by taking a walk instead.

> **SIDE BAR:** I don't know about you, but some of my best revelations from God came during a run or workout. Some of my most heartfelt prayers came during a hard bike ride against the wind. Some of my calmest moments have been when I was cooking for my family during the hectic holidays. However, I cannot think of one time when I turned to junk food in times of crisis that I felt satisfied, calm, better, healed, at peace, or joyful. It only made me feel more defeated.

---

67    1 Corinthians 6:12 "'Everything is permissible for me' – but not everything is beneficial. 'Everything is permissible for me' – but I will not be mastered by anything."

Your actions encourage others to also stand firm in their convictions. It's ok to admit it's a struggle for you to do so.

**Being confident in who you are and committed to your**
***Eternal "WHY" ENCOURAGES* others.**
**But being vulnerable *INSPIRES* others.**

When you're going through "hell," don't stop, sit down, and have a picnic! KEEP GOING! It's the only way to get through it. You will be rewarded in measure to the level of your efforts, perseverance and commitment to your goal. (Galatians 6:7-9)

Include God in the areas of health, fitness, and nutrition, just as you do with other areas in your life, like work and family, and see how your life can change. Do the best you can with what is available to you, and your efforts will be blessed. God knows your heart and where your motivations lie.

A healthy lifestyle takes work, focus, discipline and perseverance EVERY SINGLE DAY. It's a choice, hence the term "lifestyle." It's not always easy, but it is always worth it. The good news is *poor health is reversible.* It's never too late to begin. Time spent on your health and spiritual growth is never time wasted.

*PRAY, EAT, AND EXERCISE*
LIKE YOUR LIFE DEPENDS ON IT
*BECAUSE IT DOES!*

# FINAL THOUGHTS

It's been a wonderful, amazing, and sometimes painful journey, but I hope I've inspired you to "endeavor to persevere" and be your healthiest self in Christ. *"Blessed is the one who perseveres under trial because, having stood the test, that person will receive the crown of life that the Lord has promised to those who love Him."* James 1:12

I'll share a little secret though—the journey never ends, but oh is it ever fun and exciting when you know your purpose and are living your *Eternal WHY!*

Sometimes it's hard and painful, sad and frustrating, but you can't experience and appreciate love without loss, joy without sorrow, hope without struggle, success without failure, health without illness, winning without defeat, courage without fear. With each peak reached, you find healing, more peace, greater joy, and increased faith. When you experience that, you won't trade any experience or challenge conquered with God for anything. You know how they say that a traumatic event bonds people together forever? Well friends, I say *LIFE*, in and of itself, is a traumatic event. As for me, I want to travel through it with my Savior and be bonded with *Him* forever!

I'm happy to help you in any way I can. If you need prayer and encouragement along the way, or specific help with fitness, nutrition, determining the right path for you, or setting realistic goals; please, reach out and contact me through my website at www.getfitwithkimtoday.com.

Live real, friends!

Yours in health,

*Kim Clinkenbeard*

**THE END!!**

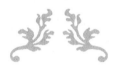

---

*"Behold, I stand at the door and knock. If anyone hears my voice and opens the door, I will come in to him and eat with him, and he with me."*

*Revelation 3:20*

---

# EXTRAS

# HEALTH QUESTIONAIRE

**"HOW DO YOU FEEL?"** Answer the following questions in each category below.

**PHYSICALLY:**

Are you tired during the day?
How is your sleep? Wake up at night & can't go back to sleep?
Have a hard time falling asleep?
Do you ache in your muscles or joints?
Headaches?
Muscle spasms?
Gas?
Bloating?
Indigestion?
Constipation?
Diarrhea?
Legs swell by end of day?
Puffy eyes & face in the morning?
Dry, brittle hair & nails?
Dry skin?
Vaginal dryness?
Hemorrhoids?
Allergies?
Sick often?
Feel "run down"?
Fatigue?
Acne?
Tooth aches?
Hot/cold flashes?
Sweating more than usual?

Trouble breathing?

Cravings- sweet & or salty?

Hungry all the time?

Hypoglycemic? (Blood sugar crashes)

Bad breath?

Body odor?

Weight gain?

**EMOTIONALLY/MENTALLY:**

Irritable?

Lack of concentration?

Brain fog?

Forgetful?

Short tempered?

Dizzy?

Unmotivated?

Exhausted?

Mood swings?

Sensitive/feelings hurt more easily?

**RELATIONALLY: (self, family, friends, co-workers)**

Negative self-talk?

Negative attitude?

Low self-esteem?

Road rage?

Overly sensitive?

Short with others?

Feelings of jealousy?

Feelings of bitterness or resentment?

Feelings of guilt or shame?

Isolating- not wanting to go out or to parties or social functions?
Sex with spouse?
Feeling disconnected?
Lonely?

## SPIRITUALLY:

Frustrated?
Not attending church?
Not doing daily quiet time?
Feel like praying isn't helping or not being answered?
Not praying? Or not consistently?
Loss of peace &/or joy?
Feeling disconnected?
Lonely?
Feelings of failure?

## "WHAT HAVE YOU DONE/NOT DONE THAT LED TO THE ABOVE"

~ rate on a scale of 1-5:
1 being "oh good grief what was I thinking?!"
And 5 being "superkalafragalisticexpialadociously awesome!" ~
Expand on each category.

**NUTRITION:** 1   2   3   4   5

**EXERCISE:** 1   2   3   4   5

**SLEEP:** 1   2   3   4   5

**STRESSES:** 1   2   3   4   5

**TRAVEL:** 1   2   3   4   5

**FUN:** 1   2   3   4   5

**SERVICE/VOLUNTEER/CHURCH:** 1  2  3  4  5

**WORK:** 1  2  3  4  5

**FAMILY/FRIENDS:** 1  2  3  4  5

# DISCLAIMER

**FITNESS. FOOD. FAITH: "Your Eternal "Why" for Everlasting Results** offers health, fitness, and nutritional information for educational, informational, and reference purposes only. This publication also includes the opinions and ideas of the author, and the information given here is designed to help you make informed decisions about your health. This book is intended to supplement, not replace, the professional medical advice, diagnosis, or treatment of health conditions from a licensed medical professional. This book is not intended to treat or diagnosis any medical health condition diagnosed, undiagnosed, treated, or untreated. Please consult your physician or other healthcare professional prior to beginning or changing any health or fitness program to ensure that it is suitable for your needs – especially if you are pregnant or have a family history of any medical concerns, illnesses, or risks.

If you have any concerns or questions about your health, you should always consult with a physician or other healthcare professional. Stop exercising immediately if you experience faintness, dizziness, pain or shortness of breath at any time. Please do not disregard, avoid, or delay obtaining medical or health-related advice from your healthcare professional because of something you may have read in this book.

All scriptures throughout this book are taken from the Holy Bible, New International Version, NIV.

# REFERENCES

1. Despres JP, Arsenault BJ, Cote M, Cartier A, Lemieux I. Abdominal obesity: the cholesterol of the 21st century? Can J Cardiol. 2008;24:7D–12D. https://www.ncbi.nlm.nih.gov/pubmed/18787730

2. Burke V. Obesity in childhood and cardiovascular risk. Clin Exp Pharmacol Physiol. 2006;33:831–837. https://www.ncbi.nlm.nih.gov/pubmed/16922816

3. Ogden CL, Yanovski SZ, Carroll MD, Flegal KM. The epidemiology of obesity. Gastroenterology.2007;132:2087–2102. https://www.ncbi.nlm.nih.gov/pubmed/17498505

4. Ogden CL, Carroll MD, Flegal KM. Epidemiologic trends in overweight and obesity. Endocrinol Metab Clin North Am. 2003;32:741–760. vii. https://www.ncbi.nlm.nih.gov/pubmed/14711060

5. Ogden CL, Carroll MD, McDowell MA, Flegal KM. Obesity among adults in the United States—no statistically significant chance since 2003-2004. NCHS Data Brief. 2007;1:1-8 https://www.ncbi.nlm.nih.gov/pubmed/19389313

6. Ogden CL, Carroll MD, Flegal KM. High body mass index for age among US children and adolescents, 2003-2006. JAMA. 2008;299:2401–2405. https://www.ncbi.nlm.nih.gov/pubmed/18505949

7. James PT. Obesity: the worldwide epidemic. Clin Dermatol. 2004;22:276–280. https://www.ncbi.nlm.nih.gov/pubmed/15475226

8. Calle EE, Thun MJ, Petrelli JM, Rodriguez C, Heath CW., Jr Body-mass index and mortality in a prospective cohort of U.S. adults. N Engl J Med. 1999;341:1097–1105. https://www.ncbi.nlm.nih.gov/pubmed/10511607

9. Field AE, Coakley EH, Must A, et al. Impact of overweight on the risk of developing common chronic diseases during a 10-year period. Arch Intern Med. 2001;161:1581–1586. https://www.ncbi.nlm.nih.gov/pubmed/11434789

10. Renehan AG, Tyson M, Egger M, Heller RF, Zwahlen M. Body-mass index and incidence of cancer: a systematic review and meta-analysis of prospective observational studies. Lancet. 2008;371:569–578. https://www.ncbi.nlm.nih.gov/pubmed/18280327

11. Peeters A, Barendregt JJ, Willekens F, Mackenbach JP, Al Mamun A, Bonneux L. Obesity in adulthood and its consequences for life expectancy: a life-table analysis. Ann Intern Med. 2003;138:24–32. https://www.ncbi.nlm.nih.gov/pubmed/12513041

12. Bamgbade OA, Rutter TW, Nafiu OO, Dorje P. Postoperative complications in obese and non-obese patients. World J Surg. 2007;31:556–560. https://www.ncbi.nlm.nih.gov/pubmed/16957821

13. Knowler WC, Barrett-Connor E, Fowler SE, et al. Reduction in the incidence of type 2 diabetes with lifestyle intervention or metformin. N Engl J Med. 2002;346:393–403. https://www.ncbi.nlm.nih.gov/pubmed/11832527

14. Neter JE, Stam BE, Kok FJ, Grobbee DE, Geleijnse JM. Influence of weight reduction on blood pressure: a meta-analysis of randomized controlled trials. Hypertension. 2003;42:878–884. https://www.ncbi.nlm.nih.gov/pubmed/12975389

15. Anderson JW, Konz EC. Obesity and disease management: effects of weight loss on comorbid conditions. Obes Res. 2001;9:326S–334S. https://www.ncbi.nlm.nih.gov/pubmed/11707561

16. Guthrie JF, Lin BH, Frazao E. Role of food prepared away from home in the American diet, 1977-78 versus 1994-96: changes and consequences. J Nutr Educ Behav. 2002;34:140–150. https://www.ncbi.nlm.nih.gov/pubmed/12047838

17. Pereira MA, Kartashov AI, Ebbeling CB, et al. Fast-food habits, weight gain, and insulin resistance (the CARDIA study): 15-year prospective analysis. Lancet. 2005;365:36–42. https://www.ncbi.nlm.nih.gov/pubmed/15639678

18. Rydell SA, Harnack LJ, Oakes JM, Story M, Jeffery RW, French SA. Why eat at fast-food restaurants: reported reasons among frequent consumers. J Am Diet Assoc. 2008;108:2066–2070. https://www.ncbi.nlm.nih.gov/pubmed/19027410

19. Stender S, Dyerberg J, Astrup A. Fast food: unfriendly and unhealthy. Int J Obes (Lond) 2007;31:887–890. https://www.ncbi.nlm.nih.gov/pubmed/17452996

20. Stender S, Dyerberg J, Astrup AV. Fast food promotes weight gain. Ugeskr Laeger. 2007;169:1804–1806. https://www.ncbi.nlm.nih.gov/pubmed/17537359

21. French SA, Jeffery RW, Forster JL, McGovern PG, Kelder SH, Baxter JE. Predictors of weight change over two years among a population of working adults: the Healthy Worker Project. Int J Obes Relat Metab Disord. 1994;18:145–154. https://www.ncbi.nlm.nih.gov/pubmed/8186811

22. French SA, Harnack L, Jeffery RW. Fast food restaurant use among women in the Pound of Prevention study: dietary, behavioral and demographic correlates. Int J Obes Relat Metab Disord. 2000;24:1353–1359. https://www.ncbi.nlm.nih.gov/pubmed/11093299

23. Stender S, Astrup A, Dyerberg J. Ruminant and industrially produced trans fatty acids: health aspects.Food Nutr Res. 2008;52 https://www.ncbi.nlm.nih.gov/pubmed/19109659

24. Mozaffarian D, Willett WC. Trans fatty acids and cardiovascular risk: a unique cardiometabolic imprint?Curr Atheroscler Rep. 2007;9:486–493. https://www.ncbi.nlm.nih.gov/pubmed/18377789

25. Willett WC, Stampfer MJ, Manson JE, et al. Intake of trans fatty acids and risk of coronary heart disease among women. Lancet. 1993;341:581–585. https://www.ncbi.nlm.nih.gov/pubmed/8094827

26. Burger KS, Kern M, Coleman KJ. Characteristics of self-selected portion size in young adults. J Am Diet Assoc. 2007;107:611–618. https://www.ncbi.nlm.nih.gov/pubmed/17383267

27. Ledikwe JH, Ello-Martin JA, Rolls BJ. Portion sizes and the obesity epidemic. J Nutr. 2005;135:905–909. https://www.ncbi.nlm.nih.gov/pubmed/15795457

28. Dhingra R, Sullivan L, Jacques PF, et al. Soft drink consumption and risk of developing cardiometabolic risk factors and the metabolic syndrome in middle-aged adults in the community. Circulation. 2007;116:480–488. https://www.ncbi.nlm.nih.gov/pubmed/17646581

29. Malik VS, Schulze MB, Hu FB. Intake of sugar-sweetened beverages and weight gain: a systematic review. Am J Clin Nutr. 2006;84:274–288. https://www.ncbi.nlm.nih.gov/pubmed/16895873

30. Bray GA, Nielsen SJ, Popkin BM. Consumption of high-fructose corn syrup in beverages may play a role in the epidemic of obesity. Am J Clin Nutr. 2004;79:537–543. https://www.ncbi.nlm.nih.gov/pubmed/15051594

31. Vos MB, Kimmons JE, Gillespie C, Welsh J, Blanck HM. Dietary fructose consumption among US children and adults: the Third National Health and Nutrition Examination Survey. Medscape J Med.2008;10:160. https://www.ncbi.nlm.nih.gov/pubmed/18769702

32. Williamson DF, Madans J, Anda RF, Kleinman JC, Kahn HS, Byers T. Recreational physical activity and ten-year weight change in a US national cohort. Int J Obes Relat Metab Disord. 1993;17:279–286. https://www.ncbi.nlm.nih.gov/pubmed/8389337

33. Miller WC, Koceja DM, Hamilton EJ. A meta-analysis of the past 25 years of weight loss research using diet, exercise or diet plus exercise intervention. Int J Obes Relat Metab Disord. 1997;21:941–947. https://www.ncbi.nlm.nih.gov/pubmed/9347414

34. Slentz CA, Duscha BD, Johnson JL, et al. Effects of the amount of exercise on body weight, body composition, and measures of central obesity: STRRIDE—a randomized controlled study. Arch Intern Med.2004;164:31–39. https://www.ncbi.nlm.nih.gov/pubmed/14718319

35. Curioni CC, Lourenco PM. Long-term weight loss after diet and exercise: a systematic review. Int J Obes (Lond) 2005;29:1168–1174. https://www.ncbi.nlm.nih.gov/pubmed/15925949

36. Borgmeier I, Westenhoefer J. Impact of different food label formats on healthiness evaluation and food choice of consumers: a randomized-controlled study. BMC Public Health. 2009;9:184. https://www.ncbi.nlm.nih.gov/pubmed/19523212

37. Wootan MG, Osborn M. Availability of nutrition information from chain restaurants in the United States. Am J Prev Med. 2006;30:266–268. https://www.ncbi.nlm.nih.gov/pubmed/16476644

38. Liu B, Balkwill A, Spencer E, Beral V. Relationship between body mass index and length of hospital stay for gallbladder disease. J Public Health (Oxf) 2008;30:161–166. https://www.ncbi.nlm.nih.gov/pubmed/18308742

39. Anand G, Katz PO. Gastroesophageal reflux disease and obesity. Gastroenterol Clin North Am. 2010;39:39–46. https://www.ncbi.nlm.nih.gov/pubmed/20202577

40. Farrell GC, Larter CZ. Nonalcoholic fatty liver disease: from steatosis to cirrhosis. Hepatology. 2006;43:S99–S112. https://www.ncbi.nlm.nih.gov/pubmed/16447287

41. Farrell GC, Teoh NC, McCuskey RS. Hepatic microcirculation in fatty liver disease. Anat Rec (Hoboken) 2008;291:684–692. https://www.ncbi.nlm.nih.gov/pubmed/18484615

42. Cave MC, Hurt RT, Frazier TH, et al. Obesity, inflammation, and the potential application of pharmaconutrition. Nutr Clin Pract. 2008;23:16–34. https://www.ncbi.nlm.nih.gov/pubmed/18203961

43. Hurt RT, Frazier TH, Matheson PJ, et al. Obesity and inflammation: III. Curr Gastroenterol Rep.2007;9:307–308. https://www.ncbi.nlm.nih.gov/pubmed/17053832

44. Hurt RT, Frazier TH, Matheson PJ, et al. Obesity and inflammation: II. Curr Gastroenterol Rep.2007;9:306–307. https://www.ncbi.nlm.nih.gov/pubmed/17209175

45. Ziegler O, Sirveaux MA, Brunaud L, Reibel N, Quilliot D. Medical follow up after bariatric surgery: nutritional and drug issues. General recommendations for the prevention and treatment of nutritional deficiencies. Diabetes Metab. 2009;35:544–557. https://www.ncbi.nlm.nih.gov/pubmed/20152742

46. Associations of total amount and patterns of sedentary behaviour with type 2 diabetes and the metabolic syndrome: The Maastricht Study Julianne D. van der Berg1,2 & Coen D. A. Stehouwer 3,4 & Hans Bosma1,2 & Jeroen H. P. M. van der Velde 3,5,6 & Paul J. B. Willems5,6 & Hans H. C. M. Savelberg5,6 & Miranda T. Schram3,4 & Simone J. S. Sep3,4 & Carla J. H. van der Kallen3,4 & Ronald M. A. Henry3,4 & Pieter C. Dagnelie2,4,7 & Nicolaas C. Schaper2,3,4 & Annemarie Koster1,2 Received: 22 October 2015 /Accepted: 14 December 2015 # The Author(s) 2016. This article is published with open access at Springerlink.com

47. Sedentary behavior: i.e. TV viewing time and life expectancy related results. http://bjsm.bmj.com/content/46/13/927

48. Am J Prev Med. 2012 Jun;42(6):563-70. doi: 10.1016/j. amepre.2011.10.026. Obesity and severe obesity forecasts through 2030. www.ncbi.nlm.nih.gov/pubmed/22608371

49. NASM NUTRITION certification/education: food, obesity rates, nutrition, diets, vitamins/minerals. http://www.nasm.org

50. NASM CERTIFIED PERSONAL TRAINER certification/ education: fitness, weight statistics, exercise, benefits, risks. http:// www.nasm.org

51. Epsom salt: benefits, uses, how to. https://www.seasalt.com/ salt-101/epsom-salt-uses-benefits

52. Dry brushing: benefits, uses, how to. http://articles.mercola. com/sites/articles/archive/2014/02/24/

53. Patil SP, Schneider H, Schwartz AR, Smith PL. Adult obstructive sleep apnea: pathophysiology and diagnosis. Chest. 2007;132:325–337. https://www.ncbi.nlm.nih. gov/pubmed/17625094

54. Alcohol, supplements, and sleep. https://www.helpguide. org/articles/sleep/cant-sleep-insomnia-treatment.htm; https:// sleepfoundation.org/sleep-topics/melatonin-and-sleep; www.sleep. org; http://www.webmd.com/sleep-disorders/news/20130118/

55. Hormones and how they affect weight, metabolism, the body. htttps://www.metaboliceffect.com/female-hormones-estrogen/

56. Insufficient sleep is a public health problem. Causes, risks, statistics related to lack of sleep. https://www.cdc.gov/features/dssleep/index.html

57. Sleep and insomnia statistics. https://www.trendstatistics.com/health/9-fascinating-insomnia-sleep-statistics/

58. Intermittent fasting, practices, metabolism. http://www.nature.com/ijo/journal/v39/n5/full/ijo2014214a.html, http://fitness.mercola.com/sites/fitness/archive/2013/12/20/intermittent-fasting-weight-loss.aspx

59. Vitamins and minerals through diet/ muti-vitamin. http://www.health.harvard.edu/womens-health/getting-your-vitamins-and-minerals-through-diet

60. Hot peppers and health benefits http://www.everydayhealth.com/high-cholesterol/diet/hot-peppers-can-help-your-heart/ http://www.naturalnews.com/039468_hot_peppers_weight_loss_metabolism.html#. https://draxe.com/capsaicin/

61. Metabolism, foods, dieting. https://www.southdenver.com/wp-content/uploads/2012/09/web1, http://www.emedexpert.com/tips/

62. Juicing, blending, cleanses, detoxes. http://www.mayoclinic.org/healthy-lifestyle/nutrition-and-healthy-eating/in-depth/whats-the-difference-between-juicing-and-blending/art-20208966, https://www.ncbi.nlm.nih.gov/pubmedhealth/PMH0072577/, http://www.slate.com/articles/double_x/doublex/2013/11/juice_cleanses_not_healthy_not_virtuous_just_expensive.html

63. Artificial Sweeteners. http://www.cbsnews.com/news/ sweeter-than-sugar-03-08-2004/, https://medlineplus.gov/ency/ article/007492.htm, http://www.cnn.com/2013/07/15/health/ artificial-sweeteners-soda/index.html, http://articles.mercola. com/sites/articles/archive/2013/10/07/sugar-substitutes.aspx#, http://www.health.harvard.edu/blog/artificial-sweeteners-sugar-free-but-at-what-cost-201207165030, http://www.foxnews.com/ health/2013/10/29/10-reasons-to-give-up-diet-soda.html, http:// www.news-medical.net/news/20110213/Daily-diet-soda-raises-stroke-risk-by-6125-Study.aspx

64. American Heart Association and American Diabetes Association Scientific Statement: Nonnutritive Sweeteners: Current use and health perspectives. *Circulation.* 2012;126:509-519. PMID: 22777177. www.ncbi.nlm.nih.gov/ pubmed/22777177, http://circ.ahajournals.org/content/126/4/509

65. Artificial sweeteners and cancer. National Cancer Institute Fact Sheet. Last reviewed August 5, 2009. www.cancer.gov/about-cancer/causes-prevention/risk/diet/artificial-sweeteners-fact-sheet. Accessed October 21, 2015. https://www.cancer.gov/about-cancer/ causes-prevention/risk/diet/artificial-sweeteners-fact-sheet

66. Johnson RJ, Appel LJ, Brands M, et al. Dietary sugars intake and cardiovascular health: A scientific statement from the American Heart Association. *Circulation.* 2009;120:1011-1020. PMID: 19704096. https://www.ncbi.nlm.nih.gov/ pubmed/19704096

67. Malik VS, Popkin BM, Bray GA, et al. Sugar-sweetened beverages and risk of metabolic syndrome and type 2 diabetes: a meta-analysis. *Diabetes Care*. 2010;33:2477-2483. PMID: 20693348. https://www.ncbi.nlm.nih.gov/pubmed/20693348

68. US Department of Health and Human Services and US Department of Agriculture. *2015–2020 Dietary Guidelines for Americans*. 8th Edition. December 2015. https://health.gov/dietaryguidelines/2015/guidelines/ Accessed January 15, 2016.

# PICTURES

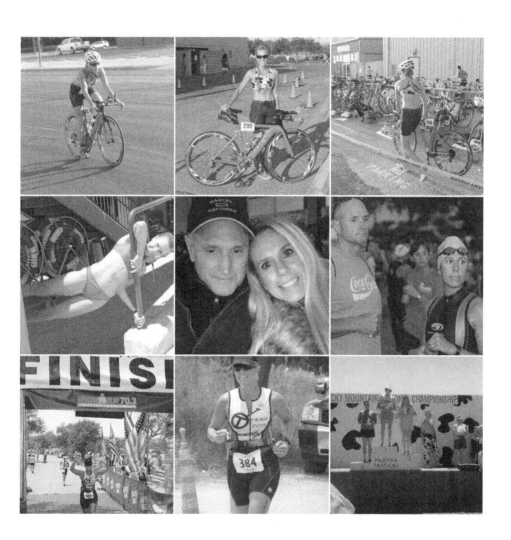

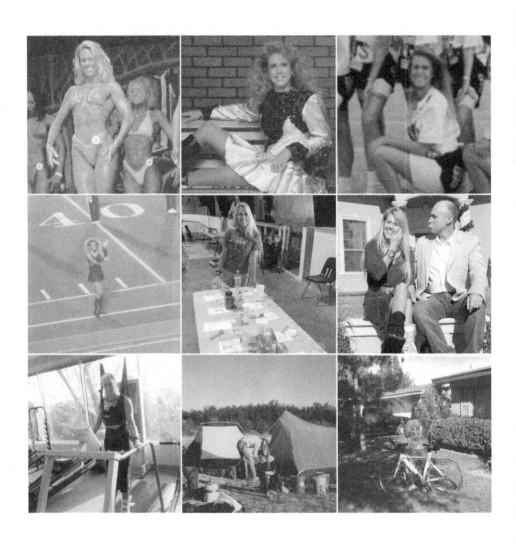

# ABOUT THE AUTHOR

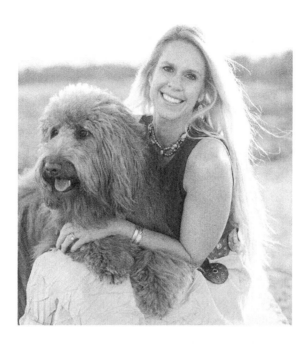

Kim is a West Texas girl through and through, still residing in her home town of Odessa with her husband and two dogs. Since 1991, she has been a leader in her community as a Fitness and Nutrition expert, with a background in twirling, dance, aerobics, figure body building, cooking, running, and 70.3 Ironman triathlons. As the owner of *Get Fit With Kim, L.L.C.,* she continues to train clients in her home gym and online.

Her healthy cooking classes have awarded her the "Best Chef of the Permian Basin" 2013, 2014, and 2016. She continues to teach both public and private cooking classes in her home, and has recently published a collection of these award-winning recipes titled, *How to Eat Pie Too! Cookbook.*

You can get your copy here: www.getfitwithkimtoday.com

It's been Kim's passion to help others achieve their fitness and health goals through personal training, group exercise, nutritional counseling and programs, healthy cooking classes, videos, writing, life coaching, and more.

Kim's philosophy is:

Get help with what you don't know. Do the best you can. Pray over the rest, and move on with life. She believes to truly be healthy, one must continue to grow in mind, body, and spirit, through healthy lifestyle changes. She is passionately committed to helping others adopt a healthier lifestyle, while ensuring they achieve their desired results through any of the services she offers.

Kim's certifications include:
NASM Certified Personal Trainer
NASM Fitness Nutrition Specialist
CrossFit Endurance Coach
USA Triathlon Coach
NASM Youth Exercise Specialist
NASM Senior Exercise Specialist
Positional Isometrics Coach
Rossiter Coach
AFAA Group Exercise Instructor
R.I.P.P.E.D. Certified Instructor
And many sub-categories

Her passion for health and love for people drives her to continue learning and sharing information. You can get her real-life tips and advice regularly on the lifestyle TV program, "Studio 7" on CBS www.cbs7.com/features/studio7, as well as through her monthly article in "Be Well Magazine." You can connect with Kim and follow her on social media sites listed below, as well as her blog, or sign-up to work with her through her website at www.getfitwithkimtoday.com. She would love to hear from you!

## Social Links

- Facebook: www.facebook.com/getfitwithkimtoday/
- Twitter: twitter.com/KimClinkenbeard
- Instagram: www.instagram.com/getfitwithkimtoday/
- You Tube: www.youtube.com/channel/ UC9ds1tSUsB7eJQEUFBuS5zA
- Linked-in: www.linkedin.com/in/

Made in the USA
Monee, IL
01 May 2023

32745175R10157